Small
Animal Medical
Differential
Diagnosis

A Book of Lists

D1260439

Small Animal Medical **Differential Diagnosis**

A Book of Lists

MARK S. THOMPSON, DVM

Diplomate, American Board of Veterinary Practitioners
Certified in Canine/Feline Practice
Brevard Animal Hospital
Brevard, North Carolina

SAUNDERS

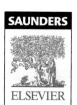

ELSEVIER

SAUNDERS
ELSEVIER

11830 Westline Industrial Drive
St. Louis, Missouri 63146

SMALL ANIMAL MEDICAL
DIFFERENTIAL DIAGNOSIS:
A BOOK OF LISTS

ISBN-13: 978-1-4160-3268-7
ISBN-10: 1-4160-3268-1

Notice

Neither the Publisher nor the Author assumes any responsibility for any loss or injury and/or damage to persons or property arising out of or related to any use of the material contained in this book. It is the responsibility of the treating practitioner, relying on independent expertise and knowledge of the patient, to determine the best treatment and method of application for the patient.

The Publisher

ISBN-13: 978-1-4160-3268-7
ISBN-10: 1-4160-3268-1

Acquisitions Editor: Anthony Winkel
Developmental Editor: Maureen Slaten
Publishing Services Manager: Patricia Tannian
Project Manager: Sarah Wunderly
Design Direction: Teresa McBryan

Working together to grow
libraries in developing countries

www.elsevier.com | www.bookaid.org | www.sabre.org

ELSEVIER | BOOK AID International | Sabre Foundation

Printed in United States

Last digit is the print number: 9 8 7 6 5 4 3 2 1

Preface

The intent of this book is to provide the veterinary clinician, intern, resident, and student with a quick, concise, and practical reference to differential diagnosis, etiology, laboratory abnormalities, and classification of clinical signs and medical disorders in dogs and cats. Although this information is readily available in full text and table form in general veterinary medical texts, it is usually scattered throughout multiple sources and is difficult to find when it is most needed. By covering hundreds of clinical signs and disorders relevant to small animal medical practice, this pocket-sized, rapid reference will help the clinician make more reliable on-the-scene decisions and allow students to more fully participate in clinical rounds with their instructors.

When Dr. Tony Winkel of Elsevier first came to me with the idea for this book, I envisioned a text that would help the veterinary student or new veterinarian when considering a differential diagnosis. However, I found myself referring to the manuscript often to help me remember some of the more esoteric rule-outs on the differential list. After 21 years in this profession, I find it easy to come up with the first six differentials, but the next four are more elusive. Thus, this book can serve the inexperienced and the experienced alike.

Small Animal Medical Differential Diagnosis is patterned after a very successful reference in human medicine titled *Handbook of Differential Diagnosis in Internal Medicine: Medical Book of Lists* by Greenberger, et al. Now in its fifth edition, this book contains lists pertaining to differential diagnosis and diagnostic criteria.

Much of the information in *Small Animal Medical Differential Diagnosis* has been distilled from other Elsevier veterinary references, especially Ettinger's *Textbook of Veterinary Internal Medicine*, sixth edition, and Nelson and Couto's *Small Animal Internal Medicine*, third edition. *Kirk and Bistner's Handbook of Veterinary Procedures and Emergency Treatment*, eighth edition, by Ford and Mazzaferro, *Small Animal Clinical Diagnosis by Laboratory Methods*, fourth edition, by Willard and Tvedten, and *Infectious Diseases of the Dog and Cat*, third edition, by Greene were also consulted frequently. The reader is encouraged to consult these texts for more detailed information.

This manual is divided into three parts featuring approximately 350 lists. Part One contains lists of differential diagnoses based on clinical signs of disease that may be identified by the clinician. Lists for more than 80 clinical signs are provided. Part Two approaches differential diagnosis from a systems perspective. Relevant lists are provided for medical conditions from 14 body systems. Part Three is an alphabetical listing of laboratory tests and values relevant to canine and feline medical diagnosis. Nearly 100 of the most common laboratory tests are featured. In all three parts, an attempt has been made to prioritize lists from most common to least common.

Acknowledgments

I would like to thank John Dodam, DVM, Diplomate American College of Veterinary Anesthesia, for his help on the topic of arterial and venous blood gases. I wish also to thank the veterinarians with whom I have worked at Brevard Animal Hospital: Dr. Christine Weaver, Dr. Clyde Brooks, and Dr. Robin Knox. Our discussions about cases often served to generate topics for this book.

Mark S. Thompson DVM, DABVP

*To my wife Sandi
and my sons Zac and Andy,
who inspire me to do things
I would not do otherwise*

Contents

Part Two

SYSTEMIC APPROACH TO DIFFERENTIAL DIAGNOSIS, 67

Section I
Cardiopulmonary Disorders, 68

Section II
Dermatologic Disorders, 90

PART ONE

Clinical Signs Approach to Differential Diagnosis

Abdominal Distension

ORGANOMEGALY

Hepatomegaly (infiltrative, inflammatory, lipidosis, neoplasia)

Splenomegaly (infiltrative, inflammatory, neoplasia, hematoma)

Renomegaly (neoplasia, infiltrative)

Miscellaneous neoplasia

Granuloma (e.g., pythiosis)

Pregnancy

FLUID

Contained in Organs

Congestion resulting from splenic torsion or volvulus, or hepatic congestion from right-sided heart failure

Cysts (paraprostatic, perinephric, hepatic)

Hydronephrosis

Distended urinary bladder

Obstruction of intestines or stomach

Ileus

Pyometra

Free Fluid in Abdomen

Transudate (portal hypertension, right-sided heart failure, hypoproteinemia secondary to protein-losing enteropathy, protein-losing nephropathy, or hepatic failure)

Modified transudate (neoplasia, postsinusoidal portal hypertension, right-sided heart failure, heartworm caval syndrome, liver disease)

Exudate (pancreatitis, feline infectious peritonitis, urine, bile, neoplasia, bowel perforation, foreign body)

Chyle (trauma, neoplasia, infection, right-sided heart failure)

Blood (coagulopathy, trauma, neoplasia)

GAS

Contained in organs

Gastric dilatation/volvulus

Intestines secondary to obstruction

Parenchymal organs infected with gas-producing bacteria

Free in abdomen

Iatrogenic (after laparoscopy, laparotomy)

Rupture of gastrointestinal tract or uterus

FAT
Obesity/lipoma

WEAKENED ABDOMINAL MUSCULATURE
Hyperadrenocorticism

FECES
Obstipation/megacolon

Abdominal Effusions and Ascites

TRANSUDATE
Portal Hypertension
Presinusoidal or sinusoidal liver disease
Right-sided heart failure

Hypoalbuminemia
Liver failure
Protein-losing enteropathy

Glomerulopathy

MODIFIED TRANSUDATE
Postsinusoidal Portal Hypertension

Right-Sided Heart Failure
Heartworm caval syndrome
Liver disease

Neoplasia

EXUDATE
Nonseptic
Pancreatitis
Feline infectious peritonitis (FIP)
Urine
Bile
Neoplasia

Septic
Bowel perforation
Foreign body

CHYLE
Trauma
Neoplasia
Infection
Right-sided heart failure

BLOOD
Coagulopathy
Trauma
Neoplasia (hemangiosarcoma)

Abdominal Pain, Acute

GASTROINTESTINAL SYSTEM
Gastrointestinal ulceration
Foreign body
Neoplasia
Adhesions
Intestinal ischemia
Intestinal spasm

UROGENITAL SYSTEM
Lower urinary tract infection
Lower urinary tract obstruction
Nonseptic cystitis (idiopathic cystitis—cats)
Prostatitis
Uroliths/renoliths/ureterolith
Pyelonephritis
Neoplasm
Metritis
Uterine torsion (rare)
Testicular torsion
Mastitis

PANCREATITIS

SPLEEN
Rupture
Neoplasm
Infection
Torsion

PERITONEUM
Peritonitis
• Septic
• Nonseptic (e.g., uroabdomen)
Adhesions

HEPATOBILIARY
Hepatitis
Cholelithiasis or cholecystitis

MUSCULOSKELETAL

Fractures
Intervertebral disk disease
Diskospondylitis
Abscess

MISCELLANEOUS

Adrenalitis (associated with hypoadrenocorticism)
Heavy metal intoxication
Vasculopathy
- Rocky Mountain spotted fever
- Infarct

Autonomic (abdominal) epilepsy
Iatrogenic
- Misoprostol
- Bethanechol
- Postoperative pain

Aggressive Behavior

CATS

Pathophysiologic Causes of Feline Aggression

Rabies
Hyperthyroidism
Seizures (epilepsy, central nervous system
  inflammation)
Paradoxical effects of therapeutic drugs
  (e.g., benzodiazepines)
Toxins (side effects)
Cognitive dysfunction
Brain neoplasia

Species-Typical Patterns of Feline Aggression

Play
Fear
Aggression between cats in a household
Petting induced
Intermale aggression
Redirected
Status/assertiveness
Pain induced/irritable
Maternal
Territorial
Predatory

Learned
Idiopathic

DOGS
Pathophysiologic Causes of Canine Aggression
Rabies
Seizure activity
Intracranial neoplasia
Cerebral hypoxia
Neuroendocrine disturbances

Species-Typical Patterns of Canine Aggression
Dominance related
Fear related
Possessive/food related
Territorial/protective
Intraspecific (intradog)
Redirected
Conflict related
Predatory
Pain/medical/irritable
Play
Maternal/hormonal
Learned
Idiopathic

Alopecia

INFLAMMATORY ALOPECIA
Traumatic
Allergy (flea, atopy, food)
Parasitic dermatitis (flea, scabies, *Cheyletiella* spp., lice,
    chiggers, etc.)
Psychogenic dermatitis

Infectious
Pyoderma
Demodicosis
Dermatophytosis
Viral
Leishmaniasis
Malassezia spp.

Immune Mediated
Sebaceous adenitis
Superficial pemphigus

Alopecia areata
Erythema multiforme
Systemic lupus erythematosus (SLE), discoid lupus
    erythematosus (DLE)
Epitheliotrophic lymphoma

Atrophic
Dermatomyositis
Cutaneous vasculitis
Postvaccinal alopecia
Lymphocytic mural folliculitis
Paraneoplastic exfoliative dermatitis
Pseudopelade

NONINFLAMMATORY ALOPECIA
Hormonal
Hyperadrenocorticism
Iatrogenic Cushing's syndrome
Hypothyroidism
Sex hormone imbalance
Alopecia X
Hyperthyroidism (cat)

Canine and Feline Pinnal Alopecia

Canine Pattern Baldness

Canine Follicular Dysplasia
Tricorrhexis nodosa
Pili torti
Color mutant alopecia
Black hair follicular dysplasia

Feline Congenital/Hereditary
Alopecia universalis (Sphinx)
Congenital hypotrichosis
Hair shaft dysplasia (Abyssinian)
Follicular dysplasia (Cornish rex)
Pili torti

Other
Anagen effluvium
Telogen defluxion
Paraneoplastic alopecia
Cyclic follicular dysplasia (seasonal flank alopecia)
Postclipping alopecia
Cicatricial alopecia
Feline preauricular alopecia
Feline acquired symmetric alopecia

Anaphylaxis

VENOMS
  Insects of Hymenoptera order (bees, hornets, ants)
  Spiders (brown recluse, black widow)
  Snakes (rattlesnakes, copperheads, water moccasins)
  Lizards (Gila monster, Mexican beaded lizard)

DRUGS
  Antibiotics (penicillins, sulfonamides, lincomycin,
    cephalosporins, aminoglycosides, tetracyclines,
    chloramphenicol, polymyxin B, doxorubicin)
  Vaccines
  Allergen extracts
  Blood products
  Parasiticides (dichlorophen, levamisole, piperazine,
    dichlorvos, diethylcarbamazine, thiacetarsamide)
  Anesthetics/sedatives (acepromazine, ketamine, barbiturates,
    lidocaine, narcotics, diazepam)
  Nonsteroidal antiinflammatory drugs (NSAIDs)
  Hormones (insulin, corticotropin, vasopressin, parathyroid
    hormone, betamethasone, triamcinolone)
  Aminophylline
  Asparaginase
  Iodinated contrast media
  Neostigmine
  Amphotericin B
  Enzymes (trypsin, chymotrypsin)
  Vitamins (vitamin K, thiamine, folic acid)
  Dextrans and gelatins

FOODS
  Milk, egg white, shellfish, legumes, citrus fruits, chocolate,
    grains

PHYSICAL FACTORS
  Cold, heat, exercise

Anuria and Oliguria

PRERENAL AZOTEMIA
  Dehydration/hypovolemia

ACUTE RENAL FAILURE

One third of cases are anuric, one third are oliguric, and one third are nonoliguric; more likely to be oliguric/anuric with severe renal toxicosis.

Toxic: exogenous, endogenous, drugs

Infectious: pyelonephritis, leptospirosis, infectious canine hepatitis, sepsis

Ischemia: progression of prerenal azotemia, vascular disease (avulsion, thrombosis, stenosis)

Immune mediated: acute glomerulonephritis, systemic lupus erythematosus (SLE), transplant rejection

Neoplasia: lymphoma

Systemic disease with renal manifestations
- Infections (feline infectious peritonitis, borreliosis, babesiosis, leishmaniasis, bacterial endocarditis)
- Pancreatitis
- Sepsis
- Multiple organ failure
- Disseminated intravascular coagulation (DIC)
- Heart failure
- SLE
- Hepatorenal disease
- Malignant hypertension
- Hyperviscosity (multiple myeloma, polycythemia vera)

POSTRENAL AZOTEMIA

Obstruction (may appear similar to anuria/oliguria)

Anxiety and Phobias

FEARS AND PHOBIAS

Fear: apprehension associated with the presence of an object, individual, or object; may be normal or abnormal, depending on context.

Phobia: quickly developed, immediate, profound abnormal response to a stimulus leading to catatonia or panic.

People

Babies, children, elderly

People in uniform

People that appear different than family members
- Color, height, facial hair

Disabled people

Men or women, depending on circumstance

Animals
    Same species
    Other species

Noise
    Especially gunshots, fireworks, thunder

Places

ANXIETY
    Separation Anxiety
        Initiators
            Change in owner's routine
            Owner returning to school or work
            Move to new home
            Visit to new environment
            After stay in kennel
            New baby, new pet
            Medical, cognitive

        Common Features of Separation Anxiety
            Hyperattached to owner
            Signs of anxiety as owner leaves
            Problems manifest when owners absent or when pet
                unable to gain access to owners
            Problem behavior begins shortly after owner leaves
            May even occur during short absences
            Pet shows exuberant greeting behavior

    Generalized Anxiety
        Poorly socialized, nervous pet

Ascites

See **Abdominal Effusions and Ascites.**

Ataxia and Incoordination

FOREBRAIN DISEASE
Typically, mild ataxia and other neurologic signs predominate.
    Generalized disease: generalized ataxia
    Unilateral disease: contralateral conscious proprioceptive
    deficits, mild gait disturbance

Postictal paraparesis: transient in nature
Paraparesis may be a side effect of anticonvulsant therapy (especially potassium bromide).

BRAIN STEM
Hemiparesis or tetraparesis; lesions severe enough to cause paralysis usually result in respiratory arrest.
Vestibular nuclei may be affected, causing vestibular ataxia, head tilt, and nystagmus; distinguish central vestibular disease from peripheral vestibular disease by presence of ipsilateral conscious proprioceptive deficits.

PERIPHERAL VESTIBULAR DISEASE
Generalized ataxia accompanied by head tilt, rotary or horizontal nystagmus, positional strabismus, and oculovestibular eye movements
Conscious proprioceptive deficits absent

CEREBELLUM
Lesions cause dysmetria, usually hypermetria.
Unilateral lesions cause ipsilateral signs.

CERVICAL SPINAL CORD
May cause forelimb monoparesis (lesions affecting spinal segments C6-T2), hemiparesis, tetraparesis; may progress to paralysis

THORACIC (T3-L3) SPINAL CORD
Mild to marked rear limb ataxia, paraparesis, paraplegia, monoparesis, or monoplegia
Rear limb reflexes exaggerated
Reduced to absent panniculus reflex caudal to lesion

LUMBOSACRAL (L4-S2) SPINAL CORD
Mild to marked rear limb ataxia, paraparesis, paraplegia, monoplegia
Reduced to absent rear limb reflexes
May see bladder and anal sphincter hypotonia

PERIPHERAL NERVE
Mild to marked ataxia, paresis, paralysis of one or more limbs
Degenerative, inflammatory, toxic, traumatic neuropathies
Hyporeflexia usually seen
Paresis or paralysis of muscle or muscles innervated by affected nerve

Blindness

CORNEAL LESIONS

Edema (trauma, glaucoma, immune-mediated keratitis such
as keratouveitis caused by canine adenovirus-1,
endothelial dystrophy, neurotropic keratitis)

Exposure keratitis

Cellular infiltrate (bacterial, viral, fungal)

Dystrophies (lipid, genetic)

Fibrosis (scar)

AQUEOUS HUMOR LESIONS

Fibrin (anterior uveitis: many causes)

Hyphema (trauma, blood-clotting deficiencies, neoplasia)

LENS LESIONS

Cataracts (genetic, metabolic/diabetic, nutritional,
traumatic, toxic)

VITREOUS HUMOR LESIONS

Hemorrhage (trauma, systemic hypertension, clotting
deficiency, neoplasia, retinal detachment)

Hyalitis (numerous infectious diseases such as feline
infectious peritonitis, penetrating injury causing cellular
infiltrate)

RETINAL LESIONS

Glaucoma

Sudden acquired retinal degeneration (SARD)

Progressive retinal atrophy

Central progressive retinal atrophy

Toxicity (fluoroquinolone administration in cats)

Retinal detachment
- Exudative/transudative (systemic hypertension, mycoses,
  viral, bacterial, fungal)
- Neoplasia
- Retinal dysplasia
- Hereditary/congenital (e.g., Collie eye anomaly)

FAILURE TO TRANSMIT VISUAL MESSAGE

Viral infections (canine distemper, feline infectious
peritonitis [FIP])

Systemic and ocular mycoses (blastomycosis, cryptococcosis,
histoplasmosis, coccidioidomycosis)

Neoplasia

Traumatic avulsion of optic nerve (traumatic proptosis)

Granulomatous meningoencephalitis

Hydrocephalus

Optic nerve hypoplasia
Immune-mediated optic neuritis

FAILURE TO INTERPRET VISUAL MESSAGE
Canine distemper virus
Feline infectious peritonitis (FIP)
Granulomatous meningoencephalitis
Systemic mycoses
Trauma
Heat stroke
Hypoxia
Hydrocephalus
Hepatoencephalopathy
Neoplasia
Storage diseases
Postictal
Meningitis

Bradycardia, Sinus

Normal variation (fit animal)
Hypothyroidism
Hypothermia
Drugs (tranquilizers, anesthetics, β-blockers, calcium entry
    blockers, digitalis)
Increased intracranial pressure
Brain stem lesion
Severe metabolic disease (e.g., uremia)
Ocular pressure
Carotid sinus pressure
High vagal tone
Sinus node disease

Cachexia and Muscle Wasting

CACHEXIA
Certain chronic disease processes stimulate the release of cyto-
kines that suppress appetite and stimulate hypercatabolism.
Cardiac disease
End-stage renal disease
Chronic infection
Chronic fever
Chronic inflammation
Neoplasia

MUSCLE WASTING

Endocrine Disease
Hyperadrenocorticism
Hyperthyroidism
Hyperparathyroidism

Starvation
Underfeeding
Poor-quality feed
Competition for food
Dental disease

Impaired Ability to Use or Retain Nutrients
Maldigestion
Malabsorption
Parasitism
Histoplasmosis
Exocrine pancreatic insufficiency
Diabetes mellitus
Protein-losing nephropathy or gastroenteropathy

Inflammatory Myopathies
Masticatory myositis
Dermatomyositis
Canine idiopathic polymyositis
Feline idiopathic polymyositis

Protozoal Myositis
Toxoplasma gondii
Neospora caninum

Inherited Myopathies
Muscular dystrophy
Hereditary Labrador retriever myopathy

Neurologic Disorders
Spinal and peripheral neuropathies
Disuse atrophy

Compulsive Behavior Disorders

COMPULSIVE DISORDERS IN DOGS
Locomotor
Spinning or tail chasing
Stereotypic pacing/circling/jumping

Fixation; staring/barking/freezing/scratching
Chasing lights, reflections, shadows
Barking; intense/rhythmic/difficult to interrupt
Head bob/tremor/head shaking
Attacking food bowl, attacking inanimate objects

Apparent Hallucinatory
Air biting or fly snapping
Staring, freezing, startled
Star/sky gazing

Self-Injurious or Self-Directed
Tail attacking, mutilation, growl/attack legs or rear
Face rubbing/scratching
Acral lick dermatitis, licking/chewing/barbering
Nail biting
Flank sucking
Checking rear

Oral
Sucking/licking
Pica, rock chewing
Polydipsia/polyphagia
Licking of objects/owners

COMPULSIVE DISORDERS IN CATS
Locomotor
Skin ripple/agitation/running, feline hyperesthesia
Circling
Freezing
Excessive/intense chasing of imaginary objects
Excessive vocalization/howling

Apparent Hallucinatory
Staring at shadows/walls
Startle
Avoiding imaginary objects

Self-Injurious or Self-Directed
Tail attacking, mutilation, growl/attack legs or rear
Face scratching/rubbing
Chewing/licking/barbering/overgrooming
Nail biting
Hyperesthesia

Oral
Wool sucking
Pica

Polydipsia/polyphagia
Licking of objects/owners

Constipation

DIETARY CAUSES
Excessive fiber in dehydrated patient
Ingestion of hair, bones, indigestible materials

COLONIC OBSTRUCTION
Deviation of rectal canal: perineal hernia
Intraluminal or intramural disorders
- Tumor
- Granuloma
- Cicatrix
- Rectal foreign body
- Congenital stricture

Pseudocoprostasis
Extraluminal disorders
- Tumor
- Granuloma
- Abscess
- Healed pelvic fracture
- Prostatomegaly
- Prostatic or paraprostatic cyst
- Sublumbar lymphadenopathy

BEHAVIORAL OR ENVIRONMENTAL CAUSES
Change in routine
Soiled or absent litter box
Refusal to defecate in house
Inactivity

DRUGS
Opiates
Anticholinergics
Sucralfate
Barium

REFUSAL TO DEFECATE
Pain in rectal or perineal area
Inability to posture to defecate
Orthopedic or neurologic problem

COLONIC WEAKNESS
   Systemic Disease
      Hypercalcemia
      Hypokalemia
      Hypothyroidism
      Chagas' disease

   Localized Neuromuscular Disease
      Spinal cord disease
      Pelvic nerve damage
      Dysautonomia
      Chronic dilatation of colon/irreversible stretching of
         colonic musculature

MISCELLANEOUS CAUSES
   Severe dehydration
   Idiopathic megacolon (cats)

Coughing

DISORDERS OF UPPER AIRWAY
   Inflammatory
      Pharyngitis
      Tonsillitis
      Tracheobronchitis
      Chronic bronchitis
      Allergic bronchitis
      Bronchiectasis
      Collapsed trachea
      Oslerus osleri infection

   Neoplastic
      Mediastinal
      Laryngeal
      Tracheal

   Allergic
      Bronchial asthma

   Other
      Bronchial compression: left atrial enlargement, hilar
         lymphadenopathy
      Foreign body
      Inhalation

DISORDERS OF LOWER RESPIRATORY TRACT

Inflammatory

Pneumonia

Bacterial
Viral: canine distemper virus
Fungal: blastomycosis, histoplasmosis,
    coccidioidomycosis
Protozoal: toxoplasmosis, pneumocystis pneumonia

Granuloma, Abscess

Chronic Pulmonary Fibrosis

Parasitic Disease

Heartworm disease *(Dirofilaria immitis)*
Lungworm disease (*Aelurostrongylus abstrusus*—cat;
    Paragonimus kellicotti—dog, cat; *Capillaria aerophilia*—
    dog, cat; *Filaroides hirthi*—dog; *Crenosoma vulpis*—dog;
    Angiostrongylus vasorum—dog)

Neoplasia

Primary or metastatic
Lymphoma

Cardiovascular

Left-sided heart failure: pulmonary edema
Pulmonary thromboembolism

Noncardiogenic Pulmonary Edema

Allergic

Eosinophilic pneumonitis
Eosinophilic pulmonary granulomatosis
Pulmonary infiltrate with eosinophils (PIE)

Other

Lung lobe torsion
Systemic bleeding disorder
Pleural effusion
Neoplasia of chest wall

Cyanosis

CENTRAL CYANOSIS
Cardiac
Intracardiac
Tetralogy of Fallot
Atrial or ventricular septal defect with pulmonic
stenosis or pulmonary hypertension

Extracardiac
Pulmonary arteriovenous fistulas
Patent ductus arteriosus (reversed)

Pulmonary
Hypoventilation
Pleural effusion
Pneumothorax
Respiratory muscle failure (fatigue, neuromuscular
disease)
Anesthetic overdose
Primary neurologic disease

Obstruction
Laryngeal paralysis
Foreign body in airway
Mass lesion of large airway (neoplasia, parasitic,
inflammatory)
Low oxygen concentration of inspired air (high
altitude, anesthetic complications)

Ventilation-Perfusion Mismatch
Pulmonary thromboembolism
Pulmonary infiltrate (edema, inflammation,
neoplasia)
Acute respiratory distress syndrome (chronic
obstructive pulmonary disease, fibrosis)

Methemoglobinemia

PERIPHERAL CYANOSIS
Central cyanosis (heart failure)
Decreased arterial supply
Peripheral vasoconstriction (hypothermia, shock)
Arterial thromboembolism
Low cardiac output
Obstruction of venous drainage
- Tourniquet or foreign object (e.g., rubber band)

- Venous thrombosis
- Right-sided heart failure

Deafness

CONGENITAL SENSORINEURAL DEAFNESS
Inherited
Many breeds of dogs
- Dalmatians
- Merle or dapple coat patterns in Collies, Shetland Sheepdogs, Great Danes, Dachshunds
- Piebald pattern in Dalmatians, Bull Terriers, Great Pyrenees, Sealyham Terriers, Greyhounds, Bulldogs, and Beagles)
- Many other dog breeds affected
White cats with blue irides and white coloration in some breeds of dogs

CONGENITAL ACQUIRED SENSORINEURAL DEAFNESS
In utero exposure to bacteria, ototoxic drugs, low oxygen tensions, or trauma

ACQUIRED LATE-ONSET CONDUCTIVE DEAFNESS
Lack of transmission of sound through tympanic membrane and auditory ossicles
Otitis externa/media
Otic neoplasia
Polyps
Trauma-induced fluid accumulation in middle ear
Atresia of tympanum or ossicles
Fused ossicles
Stenosis of ear canal leading to accumulation of fluid in middle ear

ACQUIRED LATE-ONSET SENSORINEURAL DEAFNESS
Presbycusis (age-related hearing loss)
Ototoxicity
Chronic exposure to loud noise
Hypothyroidism
Trauma
Bony neoplasia

Diarrhea, Acute

DIET
Intolerance/allergy
Rapid dietary change
Bacterial food poisoning
Dietary indiscretion

PARASITES
Helminths
Protozoa (*Giardia, Tritrichomonas,* Coccidia spp.)

INFECTIONS
Viral (parvovirus, coronavirus, feline leukemia virus [FeLV], feline immunodeficiency virus [FIV], canine distemper virus, rotavirus)
Bacterial (*Salmonella* spp., *Clostridium perfringens, Escherichia coli, Campylobacter jejuni, Yersinia enterocolitica,* other bacteria)
Rickettsial
• Salmon poisoning

OTHER CAUSES
Hemorrhagic gastroenteritis
Intussusception
Irritable bowel syndrome
Toxins (chemicals, heavy metals, toxic plants)
Drugs (antibiotics, cancer chemotherapeutic agents, anthelmintics, NSAIDs, digitalis, lactulose)
Pancreatitis
Hypoadrenocorticism

Diarrhea, Chronic

SMALL BOWEL DIARRHEA
Food intolerance or allergy
Inflammatory bowel disease
Gastrointestinal lymphoma
Pancreatic exocrine insufficiency
Chronic parasitism (hookworm, *Giardia*)
Histoplasmosis
Intestinal lymphangiectasia
Partial obstruction
Chronic intussusception
Small intestinal bacterial overgrowth
Pythiosis

LARGE BOWEL DIARRHEA
    Food intolerance or allergy
    Parasitism (whipworm, *Giardia, Tritrichomonas*)
    Clostridial colitis
    Irritable bowel syndrome
    Histoplasmosis
    Pythiosis
    Inflammatory bowel disease
- Lymphocytic-plasmacytic colitis
- Eosinophilic colitis
- Chronic ulcerative colitis
- Histiocytic ulcerative colitis (boxers)

    Neoplasia (lymphoma, adenocarcinoma)
    FeLV/FIV (infections secondary to these viruses)

Dyschezia

See **Tenesmus and Dyschezia.**

Dysphagia

ORAL LESIONS
    Fractured bones or teeth
    Periodontitis
    Trauma (laceration, hematoma)
    Feline odontoclastic resorptive lesions (caries)
    Osteomyelitis
    Retrobulbar abscess/inflammation
    Temporal-masseter myositis
    Stomatitis, glossitis, pharyngitis, gingivitis, tonsillitis, sialoadenitis
- Immune-mediated disease
- Feline herpesvirus, calicivirus, leukemia virus, immunodeficiency virus
- Lingual foreign bodies or granulomas
- Tooth root abscess
- Uremia
- Caustic chemicals

    Esophageal stricture/foreign object
    Esophagitis
    Electric cord burns

Neoplasia (malignant or benign)
Eosinophilic granuloma
Foreign object (oral, pharyngeal, laryngeal)
Sialocele
Nasophayngeal polyp

NEUROMUSCULAR DISEASE

Myasthenia gravis
Acute polyradiculitis
Masticatory myositis
Tick paralysis
Botulism
Polymyositis
Temporomandibular joint disease
Rabies
Trigeminal nerve paralysis or neuritis
Neuropathies of cranial nerves VII, IX, X, and XII
Brain stem disease
Tetanus

Dyspnea

INSPIRATORY DYSPNEA
Nasal Obstruction

Rhinitis
- Viral: feline herpesvirus, feline calicivirus, canine distemper virus
- Bacterial
- Fungal: aspergillosis, cryptococcosis, penicilliosis, rhinosporidiosis

Neoplasia: adenocarcinoma, squamous cell carcinoma, fibrosarcoma, osteosarcoma, chondrosarcoma, lymphoma, transmissible venereal tumor
Stenotic nares
Thick nasal discharge of any etiology

Pharyngeal or Laryngeal Disease

Elongated soft palate, everted laryngeal saccules
Neoplasia/mass, abscess, granuloma, extraluminal mass
Nasopharyngeal polyp
Foreign body
Laryngeal paralysis, acute/obstructive laryngitis, laryngeal collapse, laryngeal trauma

Extrathoracic Trachea
Collapsing trachea
Tracheal hypoplasia
Tracheal trauma/stricture, foreign body, neoplasia

EXPIRATORY OR MIXED DYSPNEA
Intrathoracic Trachea and Bronchi
Collapsing trachea or main-stem bronchus
Trauma, stricture, foreign body, neoplasia

Pulmonary Parenchymal Disease
Pneumonia (viral, bacterial, fungal, protozoal, aspiration)
Pulmonary edema
Pulmonary thromboembolism
Bronchial asthma
Chronic obstructive lung disease

Parasites/Severe Infestations/Heartworm, Lungworms
Pulmonary fibrosis
Neoplasia

Pleural Space Disease
Pleural effusion
Pneumothorax

Noncardiopulmonary Disease
Severe anemia
Hypovolemia
Acidosis
Hyperthermia
Neurologic disease

Dysuria

See **Stranguria, Dysuria, and Pollakiuria.**

Ecchymoses

See **Petechiae and Ecchymoses.**

Edema

INCREASED HYDROSTATIC PRESSURE
Impaired Venous Return
Congestive heart failure
Constrictive pericarditis
Ascites (cirrhosis)
Venous obstruction or compression (thrombosis, external pressure, extremity inactivity)

Small-Caliber Arteriolar Dilatation
Heat
Neurohumoral dysregulation

REDUCED PLASMA OSMOTIC PRESSURE
Hypoproteinemia
Cirrhosis (ascites)
Malnutrition
Protein-losing enteropathy
Protein-losing glomerulonephropathy (nephrotic syndrome)

LYMPHATIC OBSTRUCTION
Various inflammatory causes
Neoplasia
Postsurgical
After radiation therapy

SODIUM RETENTION
Excessive dietary intake with renal disease
Renal hypoperfusion
Increased renin-angiotension-aldosterone secretion

INFLAMMATION
Acute and chronic
Angiogenesis

Epistaxis

SYSTEMIC CAUSES
Thrombocytopenia
- Decreased production of thrombocytes (infectious, myelophthisis secondary to neoplasia, drugs, immune-mediated phenomena)

- Increased destruction (immune mediated, microangiopathy)
- Increased consumption (disseminated intravascular coagulation, vasculitis, hemorrhage)

Thrombocytopathia
- Primary (von Willebrand's disease)
- Secondary (uremia, ehrlichiosis, multiple myeloma, drugs such as NSAIDs)

Coagulation factor defects (e.g., hemophilia A and B)

Acquired coagulopathies (anticoagulant rodenticides, hepatic failure)

Increased capillary fragility (hypertension, hyperviscosity syndromes, hyperlipidemia, thromboembolic disease)

LOCAL CAUSES

Neoplasia (nasal adenocarcinoma, lymphoma, benign polyps)

Bacterial infection (usually secondary; rarely, *Bordetella, Pasteurella,* or *Mycoplasma* can be primary cause of epistaxis)

Fungal rhinitis (*Aspergillus, Cryptococcus* spp.)

Dental disease with oronasal fistulation

Nasal parasites: *Pneumonyssus caninum* (nasal mite), *Eucoleus boehmi* (formerly *Capillaria* spp.), *Cuterebra* spp.

Eosinophilic and lymphoplasmacytic rhinitis (uncommon)

Arteriovenous malformations

Failure to Grow/Failure to Thrive

SMALL STATURE AND POOR BODY CONDITION

Dietary insufficiency

Underfeeding

Poor-quality diet

Gastrointestinal disease
- Parasitism
- Inflammatory bowel disease
- Obstruction (foreign body, intussusception)
- Histoplasmosis

Hepatic dysfunction
- Portovascular anomaly
- Hepatitis
- Glycogen storage disease

Cardiac disorder
- Congenital anomaly

- Endocarditis

Pulmonary disease

Esophageal disease
- Megaesophagus
- Vascular ring anomaly

Exocrine pancreatic insufficiency

Renal disease

Renal failure (congenital or acquired)
- Glomerular disease
- Pyelonephritis

Inflammatory disease

Hormonal disease
- Diabetes mellitus
- Hypoadrenocorticism
- Diabetes insipidus
- Juvenile hyperparathyroidism

SMALL STATURE AND GOOD BODY CONDITION

Chondrodystrophy

Hormonal disease
- Congenital hypothyroidism
- Congenital hyposomatotropism (pituitary dwarfism)
- Hyperadrenocorticism

Fever of Unknown Origin

INFECTION

Bacterial

Abscessation (inapparent subcutaneous, stump pyometra, liver, pancreas)

Pyelonephrititis

Diskospondylitis

Prostatitis

Peritonitis

Pyothorax

Septic arthritis

Bartonellosis

Mycoplasma haemofilis (formerly *Hemobartonella felis*)

Borreliosis

Bacterial endocarditis

Plague

Tuberculosis

Fungal
Blastomycosis
Histoplasmosis
Coccidioidomycosis

Viral
Feline immunodeficiency virus (FIV)
Feline leukemia virus (FeLV)
Feline infectious peritonitis (FIP; *Coronavirus*)

Rickettsial
Rocky Mountain spotted fever
Ehrlichiosis
Salmon poisoning

Protozoal
Toxoplasmosis
Babesiosis
Hepatozoonosis
Cytauxzoonosis
Trypanosomiasis (Chagas' disease)
Leishmaniasis

NEOPLASIA
Lymphoma
Multiple myeloma
Leukemia
Malignant histiocytosis
Necrotic solid tumors

IMMUNE MEDIATED
Polyarthritis
Vasculitis
Meningititis
Systemic lupus erythematosus (SLE)
Immune-mediated anemia
Steroid-responsive fever
Steroid-responsive neutropenia

OTHER
Hyperthyroidism
Tissue damage
Pharmacologic agents
• Tetracycline
• Penicillins
• Sulfas
Metabolic bone disease
Idiopathic

Flatulence

Dietary intolerance (high-fiber, high-protein, or high-fat foods; high-sulfur diets; spoiled food; food change)
Maldigestion
- Exocrine pancreatic insufficiency
- Lactose intolerance

Malabsorption
Motility disorders (disrupt passage of gas)
Aerophagia
Behavior (aerophagia associated with competitive eating habits)
Various gastrointestinal disorders

Gagging

NUTRITIONAL
Food texture
Food size

INFECTIOUS
Viral encephalitis (rabies, pseudorabies)
Fungal (focal, systemic)
Bacterial encephalitis

TOXIC
Chemical (caustic chemicals, smoke)
Botulism

DEVELOPMENTAL
Cleft palate
Hydrocephalus
Achalasia

DEGENERATIVE
Laryngeal paralysis
Muscular dystrophy
Myasthenia gravis
Neuropathy of cranial nerves V, VII, IX, or XII

MECHANICAL
Foreign body
Styloid disarticulation

METABOLIC
Uremia
Hypocalcemia

NEOPLASIA
Tonsils, pharynx, epiglottis, glottis, inner ear, nasal, central
nervous system

TRAUMA
Tracheal rupture
Pharyngeal hematoma
Medulla or pons ischemia or edema

ALLERGIC OR IMMUNE MEDIATED
Rhinitis
Pharyngitis
Laryngitis
Asthma
Granuloma complex
Idiopathic glossopharyngitis

Halitosis

ORAL DISEASE
Periodontal disease (gingivitis, periodontitis, abscessation)
Neoplasia (melanoma, fibrosarcoma, squamous cell
carcinoma)
Foreign body
Trauma/fracture
Electric cord injury
Pharyngitis
Stomatitis

METABOLIC DISEASE
Renal failure (uremia)
Diabetic ketoacidosis

GASTROINTESTINAL DISEASE
Megaesophagus
Inflammatory bowel disease
Exocrine pancreatic insufficiency

RESPIRATORY DISEASE
Rhinitis/sinusitis
Neoplasia
Pneumonia of pulmonary abscess

DERMATOLOGIC DISEASE
Lip fold pyoderma
Eosinophilic granuloma
Pemphigus complex
Bullous pemphigoid
Lupus erythematosus
Drug eruption
Cutaneous lymphoma
Exposure to dimethyl sulfoxide (DMSO)

DIETARY
Aromatic foods (onions, garlic)
Fetid food (carrion)
Coprophagy

GROOMING BEHAVIOR
Anal sacculitis
Vaginitis/balanoposthitis
Lower urinary tract infections

Head Tilt

PERIPHERAL VESTIBULAR DISEASE
Otitis media/interna
Feline idiopathic vestibular disease
Geriatric canine vestibular disease
Feline nasopharygeal polyps
Middle ear tumor
• Ceruminous gland adenocarcinoma
• Squamous cell carcinoma
Trauma
Aminoglycoside ototoxicity
Hypothyroidism (possibly)

CENTRAL VESTIBULAR DISEASE
Trauma/hemorrhage
Infectious inflammatory disease
• Rocky Mountain spotted fever
• Feline infectious peritonitis (FIP)
• Bacterial
• Protozoal
• Mycotic
• Rickettsial
• Others

Granulomatous meningoencephalitis
Neoplasia
Vascular infarct
Thiamine deficiency
Metronidazole toxicity
Viral (canine distemper virus, FIP)
Toxic (lead, hexachlorophene)
Degenerative diseases (storage diseases, neuronopathies,
    demyelinating diseases)
Hydrocephalus

Hematemesis

ALIMENTARY TRACT LESION
Gastritis
Acute gastritis (common cause)
Hemorrhagic gastroenteritis
Chronic gastritis
Helicobacter-associated disease (uncertain significance in
    dog and cat)

Gastrointestinal Tract Ulceration/Erosion
Iatrogenic
Nonsteroidal antiinflammatory drugs (NSAIDs)
Corticosteroids
NSAIDs used in combination with corticosteroids

Infiltrative Disease
Neoplasia
Inflammatory bowel disease
Pythiosis (young dogs, southeastern United States)
Foreign body
Stress ulceration
- Hypovolemic shock
- Septic shock
- After gastric dilatation/volvulus
- Neurogenic shock
Hyperacidity
- Mast cell tumor
- Gastrinoma (rare)
Other causes
- Hepatic disease
- Renal disease
- Hypoadrenocorticism
- Inflammatory disease

Esophageal Disease (Uncommon)
Tumor
Severe esophagitis
Trauma

Bleeding Oral Lesion

Gallbladder Disease (Rare)

COAGULOPATHY
Thrombocytopenia/platelet dysfunction
Clotting factor deficiency
Disseminated intravascular coagulation (DIC)

EXTRAALIMENTARY TRACT LESION
Respiratory tract lesion
Lung lobe torsion
Pulmonary tumor
Posterior nares lesion

Hematochezia

ANAL DISEASE
Perianal fistulas
Anal sacculitis or abscess
Stricture
Neoplasia (anal sac adenocarcinoma)
Anal trauma
Perineal hernia
Foreign body

RECTAL AND COLONIC DISEASE
Proctitis
Colitis
- Idiopathic
- Inflammatory bowel disease
- Stress
- Infectious *(Campylobacter spp., Clostridium perfringens)*
- Histoplasmosis
- Pythiosis
Parvovirus
Parasites
- Whipworms
- Hookworms
- Coccidia

Neoplasia
- Rectal polyp
- Adenocarcinoma
- Lymphoma
- Leiomyoma or leiomyosarcoma

Prolapsed rectum

Mucosal trauma
- Foreign body or foreign material
- Iatrogenic (thermometers, enemas, fecal loops, rectal palpation)

Iliocecal intussusception

Hematuria

RENAL OR LOWER URINARY TRACT DISEASE
Inflammation/infection
Urolithiasis
Obstruction
Trauma
Neoplasia
Bleeding disorders
Heat stroke
Renal infarct
Granulomatous urethritis
Feline lower urinary tract disease (FLUTD)
Parasitism
Drug induced (cyclophosphamide)
Renal telangiectasia of Welsh Corgis
Renal hematuria of Weimaraners
Pseudohematuria (myoglobin, hemoglobin, drugs, dyes)

EXTRAURINARY DISEASE
Prostatic disease (infection, tumor, cyst, abscess)
Uterine disease (pyometra, proestrus, tumor, subinvolution of placental sites)
Vaginal (trauma, neoplasia)
Preputial/penile (trauma, neoplasia)

Hemoptysis

Heartworm disease
Thromboembolism
Severe heart failure

Fungal pneumonia
Neoplasia
Foreign body
Lung lobe torsion
Systemic bleeding disorder

Hemorrhage, Prolonged

See **Part Two, Section V: Differential Diagnosis for Thrombocytopenia, Platelet Dysfunction, and Coagulopathies, Inherited and Acquired.**

Horner's Syndrome

2.5% phenylephrine eye drops applied

NO PUPILLARY DILATION (ASSUME PREGANGLIONIC LESION)
Intracranial disease
First cervical to third thoracic (C1-T3) spinal myelopathy
Thoracic disease
Jugular furrow disease

PUPILLARY DILATION (ASSUME POSTGANGLIONIC LESION)
Feline leukemia virus, feline immunodeficiency virus
Otitis media
Otic mass
Idiopathic

Hyperthermia

FEVER
Exogenous pyrogens (infectious agents and their products,
inflammation or necrosis of tissue, immune complexes,
pharmacologic agents, bile acids)
Endogenous pyrogens (fever-producing cytokines)

HEAT STROKE
High ambient temperatures
Exercise
Poor ventilation
Brachycephalic conformation
Obesity

EXERCISE HYPERTHERMIA
Sustained exercise
Seizure disorders (especially prolonged or cluster seizures)
Hypocalcemic tetany (eclampsia)

PATHOLOGIC ETIOLOGIES
Lesions in or around anterior hypothalamus
Hypermetabolic disorders
Hyperthyroidism
Pheochromocytoma
Malignant hyperthermia
Halothane
Succinylcholine

Hypothermia

PREDISPOSING FACTORS
Anesthesia
Low ambient temperature
Neonate
Small size
Elderly
Sick
Debilitated
Hyperlipidemia
Pancreatitis
Constipation
Dystocia
Skin fold dermatopathies
Seborrhea
Congestive heart failure
Systemic hypertension
Shorter life span
Earlier visible signs of aging
Neoplasia (mammary cancer, transitional cell carcinoma)
Increased surgical and anesthetic risk

Icterus (Jaundice)

HEMOLYSIS
Autoimmune hemolytic anemia
Hemolytic anemia secondary to drugs, neoplasia

Infectious (*Ehrlichia canis, Babesia canis, Babesia felis, Mycoplasma hemocanis, Mycoplasma hemofelis, Cytauxzoon felis,* heartworm disease, feline leukemia virus [FELV])

Toxic (onions, lead, copper, methylene blue, benzocaine, proplylene glycol, acetaminophen [cats], phenazopyridine)

Fragmentation (disseminated intravascular coagulation, hemangiosarcoma, vena cava syndrome)

Erythrocyte membrane or enzyme defects (pyruvate kinase deficiency [Beagle, Basenji], phosphofructokinase deficiency [English Springer Spaniel], stomatocytosis of chondrodysplastic Malamutes)

Congenital porphyria

HEPATOBILIARY DISEASE

Cholangiohepatitis

Chronic inflammatory hepatic disease

Cirrhosis

Diffuse neoplasia

Copper toxicity

Toxic hepatopathy (anticonvulsants, mebendazole, oxibendazole, diethylcarbamazine, inhalation anesthetics, thiacetarsamide, acetaminophen, trimethoprim-sulfa)

Hepatic lipidosis

Feline infectious peritonitis (FIP)

Idiosyncratic drug reaction

POSTHEPATIC BILIARY OBSTRUCTION

Pancreatitis

Enteritis

Trauma

Neoplasia

Calculus

Stricture

Ruptured bile duct or gallbladder

Inappropriate Elimination

DOGS

Medical Causes

Fecal House Soiling

Increased volume of feces (maldigestion, malabsorption, high-fiber diets)

Increased frequency of voiding (colitis, diarrhea)

Compromised neurologic function (peripheral nerve impairment, spinal cord disease, brain tumor, encephalitis, infection, degenerative brain disorders)

Joint pain

Sensory decline

Urinary House Soiling

Diseases causing polyuria (e.g., renal disease, hyperadrenocorticism, diabetes, pyometra)

Increased urinary frequency (urinary tract infection, urolithiasis, bladder tumors, prostatitis, abdominal masses)

Impaired bladder control (peripheral nerve disease, spinal cord disease, brain tumor, encephalitis, infection, degenerative brain disorders)

Urethral incompetence

Anatomic problems

Behavioral Causes

Inadequate training

Submissive urination

Excitement urination

Cognitive dysfunction

Marking

Separation anxiety

Management-related problems

Location or surface preference

CATS

Medical Causes

Fecal House Soiling

Increased volume of feces (maldigestion, malabsorption, high-fiber diets)

Increased frequency of voiding (colitis, diarrhea)

Compromised neurologic function (peripheral nerve impairment, spinal cord disease, brain tumor, encephalitis, infection, degenerative brain disorders)

Joint pain

Anal sacculitis

Hyperthyroidism

Neoplasia

Urinary House Soiling

Diseases causing polyuria (e.g., renal disease, hyperadrenocorticism, diabetes, pyometra)

Increased urinary frequency (feline lower urinary tract disease [FLUTD], urolithiasis, idiopathic cystitis)

Impaired bladder control (peripheral nerve disease, spinal cord disease, brain tumor, encephalitis, infection, degenerative brain disorders)

Joint pain

Hyperthyroidism

Neoplasia

Anatomic problems

Behavioral causes

Litterbox aversion

Aversive disorder (deodorant, ammonia)

Inadequate cleaning

Discomfort during elimination (FLUTD, constipation, diarrhea, arthritis)

Unacceptable litter (texture, depth, odor, plastic liner)

Unacceptable box (too small, sides too high, covered)

Disciplined, medicated, or frightened in box

Location aversion

Too much traffic

Traumatic/fearful experience in area

Other

Location preference

Surface preference

Anxiety (owner absence, high cat density, moving, new furniture, inappropriate punishment, teasing, household changes, remodeling in home)

Need for privacy (other pets, anything that makes box less accessible to cat)

Cognitive dysfunction

Incontinence, Fecal

NONNEUROLOGIC DISEASE

Colorectal Disease

Inflammatory bowel disease

Neoplasia

Constipation

Anorectal disease
Perianal fistula
Neoplasia
Surgery (anal sacculectomy, perianal herniorrhaphy, rectal resection and anastomosis)

Miscellaneous
Decreased mentation
Old age
Severe diarrhea
Irritable bowel disease

NEUROLOGIC DISEASE
Sacral Spinal Cord Disease
Diskospondylitis
Neoplasia
Degenerative myelopathy
Congenital vertebral malformation
Sacrococcygeal hypoplasia of Manx cats
Sacral fracture
Sacrococcygeal subluxation
Lumbosacral instability
Meningomyelocele
Viral meningomyelitis

Peripheral Neuropathy
Trauma
Penetrating wounds
Repair of perineal hernia
Perineal urethrostomy
Hypothyroidism
Diabetes mellitus
Dysautonomia

Incontinence, Urinary

BLADDER DISTENDED
Neurogenic
Lower motor neuron disease (sacral [S1-S3] segments or peripheral nerves)
Bladder easily expressed, dribbles urine
Upper motor neuron disease
Bladder difficult to express; may be associated with paresis, paralysis

Obstructive
Reflex dyssynergia (functional obstruction)
Mechanical obstruction (uroliths, tumors, strictures)

BLADDER NOT DISTENDED
Dysuria/Pollakiuria Absent
Urethral sphincter mechanism incompetence
(middle-aged to older spayed or neutered dogs)
Congenital (ectopic ureters, patent urachus)

Dysuria/Pollakiuria Present
Detrusor hyperreflexia/instability (uroliths, urinary tract
infection)

Infertility, Female (Canine)

NORMAL CYCLES
Improper breeding management
Infertile male
Elevated diestrual progesterone
- Early embryonic death
- Lesions in tubular system (vagina, uterus, uterine tubes)
- Placental lesions (brucellosis, herpes infection)
Normal diestrual progesterone
- Cystic follicles (ovulation failure)

ABNORMAL CYCLES
Abnormal Estrus
Will Not Copulate
Not in estrus
Inexperience
Partner preference
Vaginal anomaly
Hypothyroidism?

Prolonged Estrus
Cystic follicles
Ovarian neoplasia
Exogenous estrogens

Short Estrus
Observation error
Geriatric

Abnormal Interestrual Interval
Prolonged interval
Photoperiod (queen)
Pseudopregnant/pregnant (queen)
Normal breed variation
Glucocorticoids (bitch)
Geriatric
Luteal cysts

Short Interval
Normal (especially queen)
Ovulation failure (especially queen)
Corpus luteum failure
"Split heat" (bitch)
Exogenous drugs

NOT CYCLING
Prepubertal
Ovariohysterectomy
Estrus suppressants
Silent heat
Unobserved heat
Photoperiod (queen)
Intersex (bitch)
Ovarian dysgenesis
Hypothyroidism (possibly)
Glucocorticoid excess
Hypothalamic-pituitary disorder
Geriatric

Infertility, Male (Canine)

INFLAMMATORY EJACULATE
Prostatitis
Orchitis
Epididymitis

AZOOSPERMIA
Sperm-rich fraction not collected
Sperm not ejaculated
- Incomplete ejaculation
- Obstruction
- Prostate swelling
Sperm not produced

- Endocrine
- Testicular
- Metabolic

ABNORMAL MOTILITY/MORPHOLOGY
Iatrogenic
Prepubertal
Poor ejaculation
Long abstinence

ABNORMAL LIBIDO
Female not in estrus
Behavioral
Pain
Geriatric

NORMAL LIBIDO
Improper stud management
Infertile female

NORMAL LIBIDO/ABNORMAL MATING ABILITY
Orthopedic
Neurologic
Prostatic disease
Penile problem
Prepuce problem

Joint Swelling

Trauma
Degenerative joint disease
Neoplasia
Inflammatory joint disease—infectious
- Septic (bacterial)
- Fungal arthritis
  - Blastomycosis
  - Coccidioidomycosis
  - Cryptococcosis
- Lyme borreliosis
- Rickettsial arthritis
- Mycoplasma
- Bacterial L form–associated arthritis (cats)
- Viral arthritis (calicivirus infection—kittens)
Inflammatory joint disease—noninfectious
- *Nonerosive*

- Immune-mediated polyarthritis (idiopathic)
- Systemic lupus erythematosus (SLE)
- Breed-specific polyarthritis syndromes
- Akita, Boxer, Weimaraners, Bernese Mountain Dog, German Shorthaired Pointer, Beagle, Shar-Pei
- Lymphocytic/plasmacytic synovitis
- Drug reaction
- Chronic infection (bacterial, rickettsial, Lyme borreliosis, heartworm disease)
- *Erosive*
  - Rheumatoid arthritis
  - Erosive polyarthritis of greyhounds
  - Feline chronic progressive polyarthritis

Lameness

ORTHOPEDIC
Trauma
Fracture
Luxation, subluxation
Toenail trauma
Bone contusion

Infectious
Osteomyelitis (bacterial, fungal)

Developmental
Patellar luxation
Osteochondrosis
Panosteitis
Hypertrophic osteodystrophy
Avascular necrosis of femoral head
Nonunited anconeal process
Bone cysts

Nutritional
Vitamin D deficiency (rickets)

Neoplasia
Osteosarcoma
Multiple myeloma
Metastatic to bone

JOINT DISEASE
See **Joint Swelling**.

MUSCLES
  Trauma
    Contusion
    Strain
    Laceration
    Rupture

  Inflammatory
    Canine idiopathic polymyositis
    Feline idiopathic polymyositis
    Dermatomyositis

  Infectious
    Protozoal myositis

TENDONS
  Trauma
    Laceration
    Severance
    Avulsion

LIGAMENTS
  Trauma
    Rupture
    Tear
    Hyperextension

Lymphadenopathy (Lymph Node Enlargement)

INFILTRATIVE LYMPHADENOPATHIES
  Neoplastic
    Primary hemolymphatic (lymphoma, multiple myeloma,
      systemic mast cell disease, leukemias, malignant
      histiocytosis, lymphomatoid granulomatosis)
    Metastatic neoplasia (carcinomas, sarcomas, malignant
      melanoma, mast cell tumors)

  Nonneoplastic
    Eosinophilic granuloma complex
    Nonneoplastic mast cell infiltration

PROLIFERATIVE AND INFLAMMATORY LYMPHADENOPATHIES
  Infectious
    Bacterial
      • Localized bacterial infection

- Septicemia
- Systemic infection (e.g., *Borrelia burgdorferi, Brucella canis, Yersinia pestis, Corynebacterium, Mycobacterium, Nocardia, Streptococcus, Actinomyces, Bartonella* spp.)
- Contagious streptococcal lymphadenopathy

Parasitic (toxoplasmosis, demodicosis, babesiosis, cytauxzoonosis, hepatozoonosis, leishmaniasis, trypanosomiasis, *Neospora caninum*)

Rickettsial (ehrlichiosis, Rocky Mountain spotted fever, salmon poisoning)

Viral (feline immunodeficiency virus, feline leukemia virus, feline infectious peritonitis, canine viral enteritis, infectious canine hepatitis)

Fungal (blastomyosis, cryptococcosis, histoplasmosis, aspergillosis, coccidioidomycosis, phaeohyphomycosis, phycomycosis, sporotrichosis, others)

Algal (protothecosis)

Melena

INGESTED BLOOD
Oral lesions
Nasopharyngeal lesions
Pulmonary lesions
Diet

PARASITISM
Hookworms

NEOPLASIA
Adenocarcinoma
Lymphoma
Leiomyoma or leiomyosarcoma
Mast cell tumor
Gastrinoma

UPPER GASTROINTESTINAL INFLAMMATION
Acute gastritis
Gastroduodenal ulceration/erosion
Hemorrhagic gastroenteritis
Inflammatory bowel disease
Foreign body

DRUGS
  Nonsteroidal antiinflammatory drugs (NSAIDs)
  Glucocorticoids

MISCELLANEOUS
  Pancreatitis
  Liver failure
  Renal failure
  Hypoadrenocorticism
  Gastrointestinal ischemia (shock, volvulus, intussusception)
  Arteriovenous fistula
  Polyps
  Coagulopathies

Muscle Wasting

See **Cachexia and Muscle Wasting.**

Nasal Discharge

See **Sneezing and Nasal Discharge.**

Nystagmus

PERIPHERAL VESTIBULAR DISEASE
Horizontal nystagmus; fast phase toward normal side; no change with varying head position.
  Otitis media/interna
  Feline idiopathic vestibular disease
  Canine geriatric vestibular disease
  Neoplasia
  Granuloma
  Trauma
  Ototoxic drugs
  Neuropathy (hypothyroid, cranial nerve VIII disease)

CENTRAL VESTIBULAR DISEASE
Horizontal, vertical, or rotary nystagmus; direction may change with varying head position.
  Trauma/hemorrhage

Infectious inflammatory disease
Granulomatous meningoencephalitis
Neoplasia
Vascular infarct
Thiamine deficiency
Metronidazole toxicity
Viral (canine distemper virus, feline infectious peritonitis)
Toxic (lead, hexachlorophene)
Degenerative diseases (storage diseases, neuronopathies, demyelinating diseases)
Hydrocephalus

Obesity

CAUSES

Excessive feeding
Malnutrition
Lack of exercise
Genetic predisposition
Hypothyroidism
Hyperadrenocorticism
Hyperinsulinism
Acromegaly
Hypopituitarism
Hypothalamic dysfunction
Drugs (glucocorticoids, progestagens, phenobarbital, primidone)

HEALTH RISKS

Degenerative joint disease
Traumatic joint disease
Intervertebral disk disease
Dyspnea: Pickwickian syndrome
Heat intolerance
Exercise intolerance
Diabetes mellitus (insulin resistance)

Oliguria

See **Anuria and Oliguria.**

Pallor

ANEMIA

Regenerative Anemia

Immune-mediated hemolytic anemia (extravascular, intravascular)

Erythrocytic parasites *(Bartonella, Babesia, Cytauxzoon* spp.*)*

Fragmentation (disseminated intravascular coagulation, heartworm disease, hemangiosarcoma, vasculitis, hemolytic-uremic syndrome, diabetes mellitus)

Pyruvate kinase deficiency

Phosphofructokinase deficiency

Feline porphyria

Copper toxicity

Neonatal isoerythrolysis

Oxidative injury (onions, acetaminophen, zinc, benzocaine, mothballs, phenazopyridine)

Blood loss (external blood loss, blood loss to a body cavity, coagulopathies, endoparasites, gastrointestinal blood loss)

Nonregenerative Anemia

Anemia of chronic disease

Anemia from renal failure

Feline leukemia virus (FeLV)

Endocrine (mild anemia associated with hypoadrenocorticism, hypothyroidism)

Myeloaplasia/aplastic anemia (FeLV infection, ehrlichiosis, trimethoprim-sulfa, estrogen toxicity, phenylbutazone, chemotherapy, chloramphenicol)

Myelodysplasia

Myeloproliferative and lymphoproliferative disorders

Myelofibrosis

SHOCK

Cardiogenic

Decreased ventricular function
- Dilated cardiomyopathy
- Myocarditis
- Myocardial infarction

Compromised ventricular filling
- Hypertrophic cardiomyopathy
- Cardiac tamponade

Severe endocardiosis

Outflow obstruction

- Intracardiac tumors
- Aortic stenosis
- Hypertrophic obstructive cardiomyopathy
- Heartworm disease
- Thrombosis
- Severe arrhythmia

Noncardiogenic
   Trauma
   Hypovolemia
- Severe blood loss
- Dehydration
- Hypoadrenocorticism
   Disruptions in blood flow
- Sepsis and endotoxemia
- Hypotension

Paresis and Paralysis

UPPER MOTOR NEURON
   Tetraparesis or hemiparesis
- Severe forebrain lesion
- Brain stem lesion
- First to fifth cervical (C1-C5) spinal lesion
   Paraparesis or rear limb monoparesis
- Third thoracic to third lumbar (T3-L3) spinal lesion

LOWER MOTOR NEURON
   Tetraparesis
   Generalized lower motor neuron disease
- Flaccid paresis/paralysis
  - Acute polyradiculoneuritis/"coonhound paralysis"
  - Tick paralysis
  - Botulism
  - Myasthenia gravis
- Toxicants
  - Coral snake
  - Black widow spider
  - Herbicides (2,4 D)
  - Macadamia nuts
   Paraparesis
- Fourth lumbar to second sacral (L4-S2) spinal lesion
   Hemiparesis with lower motor neuron forelimb
- Sixth cervical to second thoracic (C6-T2) spinal lesion

Aortic thromboembolism
Degenerative myelopathy
Monoparesis
Peripheral nerve lesion

Petechiae and Ecchymoses

THROMBOCYTOPENIA
Increased Platelet Destruction
Immune-mediated thrombocytopenia
Systemic lupus erythematosus (SLE)
Heartworm disease

Decreased Platelet Production
Bone Marrow Suppression
Infectious disease (ehrlichiosis, babesiosis, Rocky
Mountain spotted fever, leishmaniasis, feline
leukemia virus, feline immunodeficiency virus)
Neoplasia
Drug reactions
Myeloproliferative disease
Virus-associated myelodysplasia
Estrogen toxicity

Consumption of Platelets
Disseminated intravascular coagulation (DIC)
Vasculitis

Sequestration of Platelets (Unlikely to Cause Clinical Signs)
Splenomegaly
Hepatomegaly
Endotoxemia

THROMBOPATHIA
Inherited
Cocker Spaniel, Otterhound, Great Pyrenees, cats

Acquired
Drugs (aspirin, cephalothin, acepromazine)
Uremia
Liver disease
Dysproteinemias

Von Willebrand's disease
> Lack of von Willebrand's factor leads to impaired platelet adhesion.

VASCULAR PURPURA
> Vasculitis secondary to infectious, inflammatory, immune-mediated, neoplasia, drug reaction, hyperadrenocorticism

Pollakiuria

See **Stranguria, Dysuria, and Pollakiuria.**

Polyuria and Polydipsia

Renal failure
Diabetes mellitus
Hyperadrenocorticism (Cushing's syndrome)
Lower urinary tract disease
- Infection
- Urolithiasis
- Neoplasia
- Anatomic problem
- Neurologic problem

Pyometra
Hypercalcemia
Hypoadrenocorticism (Addison's disease)
Pyelonephritis
Hypokalemia
Iatrogenic (corticosteroids, diuretics, anticonvulsants)
Hyperthyroidism
Hepatic insufficiency
Postobstructive
Diabetes insipidus
- Central
- Renal

Psychogenic drinking
Renal glycosuria

Pruritus

ALLERGY
Flea allergy
Atopic dermatitis
Food allergy/intolerance
Contact dermatitis
Mosquito-bite hypersensitivity
Eosinophilic plaque (cats)

PARASITES
Flea infestation
Scabies
Pediculosis (lice)
Cheyletiellosis
Chiggers
Cutaneous larval migrans
Demodicosis (often not pruritic)
Otodectic acariasis

INFECTIOUS AGENTS
Pyoderma
Malassezia dermatitis

BEHAVIORAL
Acral lick dermatosis
Psychogenic alopecia

IMMUNE-MEDIATED
Pemphigus foliaceus

DRUG ERUPTION

MISCELLANEOUS
Cornification defects
Superficial necrolytic dermatitis
Tail dock neuroma
Rhabditic dermatitis

Ptyalism (Excessive Salivation)

ORAL CAVITY DISEASE
Oral trauma (tooth fractures, mandibular fractures,
   maxillary fractures)
Severe periodontal disease

Oral masses (neoplasia, granuloma, eosinophilic granuloma)

Stomatitis (toxins, infections, immune-mediated disease, immunologic or nutritional deficiency)

Glossitis (chemical or environmental irritants, viral infections, uremia, immune-mediated disease, tumors)

Faucitis (cats)

Mucocutaneous junction lesions

Foreign body

ORAL CAVITY NORMAL

Drugs and toxins (bitter taste; insecticides such as organophosphates, pyrethrins, and D-limonene; caustic chemicals; poison toads and salamanders)

Nausea

Hepatic encephalopathy/portosystemic shunt

Seizures

Space-occupying lesions in pharynx

Cranial nerve (CN) deficits (CN V: inability to close mouth; CN VII: inability to move lip; CNs X, XI, and XII: loss of gag lesion and inability to swallow)

Rabies virus

Dysphagia

Behavior

Salivary gland hypersecretion

Regurgitation

ESOPHAGEAL DISEASE

Megaesophagus (primary or secondary)

Esophagitis

Mechanical obstruction (foreign body, vascular ring anomaly, stricture)

ALIMENTARY DISORDERS

Pyloric outflow obstruction

Gastric dilatation/volvulus

Hiatal hernia

NEUROPATHIES

Peripheral neuropathy (polyradiculitis, polyneuritis, lead poisoning, giant cell axonal neuropathy)

NEUROMUSCULAR JUNCTION ABNORMALITIES

Myasthenia gravis (focal or generalized)

Tetanus

Botulism
Acetylcholinesterase toxicity

IMMUNE-MEDIATED DISORDERS
Systemic lupus erythematosus (SLE)
Polymyositis
Dermatomyositis

ENDOCRINE DISEASE
Hypothyroidism
Hypoadrenocorticism

Seizure

EXTRACRANIAL CAUSES
Toxins (e.g., strychnine, chlorinated hydrocarbons,
    organophosphates, lead, ethylene glycol, metaldehyde)
Metabolic disease (e.g., hepatic encephalopathy,
    hypoglycemia, hypocalcemia)
Hepatic disease
Electrolyte disturbances (e.g., hypernatremia)
Severe uremia
Hyperlipoproteinemia
Hyperviscosity (multiple myeloma, polycythemia)
Hyperosmolality (diabetes mellitus)
Heat stroke

INTRACRANIAL CAUSES
See **Part Two, Section XI: Differential Diagnosis for
Inflammatory Disease of the Nervous System**.

Infectious disease
Neoplasia (primary brain tumor, lymphoma, metastatic
    tumors)
Granulomatous meningoencephalitis
Hemorrhage/infarct (renal failure, hypothyroidism,
    hyperthyroidism, hypertension, septic emboli, neoplasia,
    coagulopathies, heartworm disease, vasculitis)
Congenital malformations (lissencephaly, hydrocephalus)
Necrotizing encephalitis
Degenerative diseases (metabolic storage diseases,
    leukodystrophies, hypomyelination disorders, spongy
    disorders)

IDIOPATHIC EPILEPSY

Sneezing and Nasal Discharge

NASAL AND UPPER RESPIRATORY DISEASE
Infectious
Viral: herpesvirus, calicivirus, canine distemper virus
Fungal: *Aspergillus, Cryptococcus, Rhinosporidium,*
Penicillium spp.
Parasitic: *Pneumonyssus caninum* (nasal mite), *Eucoleus*
boehmi (formerly *Capillaria* spp.), *Cuterebra* spp.

Inflammatory
Allergic rhinitis
Lymphocytic-plasmacytic rhinitis
Acquired nasopharyngeal stenosis
Nasopharyngeal polyps

Neoplasia
Adenocarcinoma, squamous cell carcinoma
Fibrosarcoma, osteosarcoma, chondrosarcoma
Lymphoma, transmissible venereal tumor

Foreign Body

Congenital
Cleft palate
Ciliary dyskinesia

Dental Disease
Tooth root abscess
Oronasal fistula

Trauma

SYSTEMIC DISEASE
Infectious
Canine distemper virus
Canine infectious tracheobronchitis
Pneumonia

Hypertension
Hyperthyroidism
Hyperadrenocorticism
Renal disease
Pheochromocytoma

Coagulopathies
Thrombocytopenia
Vitamin K rodenticide toxicity
Rocky Mountain spotted fever

Hyperviscosity
Multiple myeloma, lymphoma

Stertor and Stridor

STERTOR
Snoring or snorting associated with partial nasal or nasopharyngeal obstruction.

Intranasal Disorders
Congenital deformities
Masses
Exudates
Clotted blood

Pharyngeal Disease
Brachycephalic airway syndrome
Elongated soft palate
Nasopharyngeal polyp
Foreign body
Neoplasia
Abscess
Granuloma
Extraluminal mass

STRIDOR
High-pitched wheeze caused by air turbulence in upper airway associated with laryngeal disease or narrowing of extrathoracic trachea.

Laryngeal Disease
Neoplasia
Polyps
Laryngeal paralysis
Laryngeal trauma
Foreign body
Acute laryngitis/obstructive laryngitis

Extrathoracic Tracheal Disease
Neoplasia
Foreign body
Extrathoracic collapsing trachea
Extraluminal mass

Stranguria, Dysuria, and Pollakiuria

STRANGURIA/POLLAKIURIA
  Small Bladder
    Cystitis
      • Infectious agents
      • Idiopathic cystitis (cats)
    Detrusor hyperspasticity
    Urethritis
    Urethral mass

  Large Bladder
    Lower urinary tract obstruction
      • Functional
      • Mechanical

URINARY RETENTION
  Easy Catheterization
    Normal Neurologic Examination
      Cystic calculi or mass
      Detrusor areflexia from overdistension
      Reflex dyssynergia

    Abnormal Neurologic Examination
      Detrusor areflexia with sphincter areflexia (lower
        motor neuron)
      Detrusor areflexia with sphincter hypertonia (upper
        motor neuron)
      Dysautonomia

  Difficult Catheterization
    Urethral spasm
    Urethral calculi
    Urethral neoplasia
    Granulomatous urethritis
    Urethral inflammation
    Prostatic disease
    Mucoid or crystalline plug (cats)

Stomatitis

Infectious disease
  • Feline immunodeficiency virus (FIV)
  • Feline leukemia virus (FeLV)

- Feline syncytium-forming virus
- Feline calicivirus
- Feline herpesvirus
- Feline infectious peritonitis (FIP)
- Bartonellosis
- Canine distemper virus
- Feline panleukopenia virus
- Candidiasis

Immunosuppressive disease
Feline eosinophilic granuloma complex
Idiopathic feline chronic gingivitis/stomatitis
Immune-mediated disease

- Systemic lupus erythematosus (SLE)
- Bullous (pemphigus) disease
- Idiopathic vasculitis
- Toxic epidermal necrolysis
- Ulcerative gingivitis/stomatitis of Maltese Terriers

Stupor and Coma

INCREASED INTRACRANIAL PRESSURE
Encephalitis
Meningitis
Neoplasia
Granulomas
Abscess
Vascular events
Trauma
Underlying metabolic injury (e.g., hypertension)

CEREBRAL EDEMA
Vasogenic (brain masses that lead to breakdown of
   blood-brain barrier)
Cytotoxic (hypoxia, neuroglycopenia)
Interstitial (hydrocephalus)

HERNIATION OF BRAIN TISSUE
Caudal transtentorial herniation
Foramen magnum herniation

Syncope

NORMAL CEREBRAL PERFUSION
Severe hypoxemia
Hypoglycemia

CEREBRAL HYPOPERFUSION
Normotension
Cerebrovascular disease
Cerebral vasoconstriction

Systemic Hypotension
Decreased Cardiac Output
Loss of Preload
Cardiac tamponade, atrial ball thrombi, atrial
myxoma, atrioventricular (AV) valve stenosis,
hypovolemia, diuretics

Obstruction to Flow
Aortic and subaortic stenosis, pulmonic stenosis,
pulmonary hypertension, pulmonary
thromboembolism, outflow tract tumors,
myocardial infarction, hypertropic and
restrictive cardiomyopathy, systolic anterior
motion of mitral valve, infundibular stenosis

Arrhythmias
Bradyarrhythmias: sick sinus syndrome,
third-degree AV block, persistent atrial
standstill, β-blockers, calcium channel blockers
Tachyarrhythmias: atrial fibrillation, atrial
tachycardia, AV reentrant tachycardia,
ventricular tachycardia, drug-induced
proarrhythmia, torsades de pointes

Loss of Vascular Resistance
Drug therapy: angiotensin-converting enzyme
(ACE) inhibitors, β-blockers, calcium channel
blockers, hydralazine, nitrates, α-blockers,
phenothiazines
Reflex syncope (neurally mediated): orthostatic,
postexertion, micturition, defecation, cough,
emotional distress, pain, carotid sinus
hypersensitivity
Autonomic nervous system disease: primary or
secondary (diabetes mellitus, paraneoplastic,

chronic renal failure, autoimmune disease, amyloidosis)

Tachycardia, Sinus

Anxiety/fear
Excitement
Exercise
Pain
Hyperthyroidism
Hyperthermia/fever
Anemia
Hypoxia
Shock
Hypotension
Sepsis
Drugs (anticholinergics, sympathomimetics)
Toxicity (e.g., chocolate, hexachlorophene)
Electric shock

Tenesmus and Dyschezia

COLONIC OR RECTAL OBSTRUCTION
Constipation
Pelvic fracture
Rectal neoplasia
Prostatomegaly
Perineal hernia
Pelvic canal mass
Rectal granuloma
Rectal foreign body
Rectal stricture

PERINEAL INFLAMMATION OR PAIN
Anal sacculitis
Perianal fistula
Perianal abscess/abscessed anal sac

RECTAL INFLAMMATION OR PAIN
Rectal tumor/polyp
Proctitis
Histoplasmosis
Pythiosis

Tremor

PHYSIOLOGIC TREMOR
Hypothermia
Heavy exercise/exhaustion

PATHOLOGIC TREMOR
Metabolic disorders (renal disease, hypoglycemia, hypocalcemia, hypoadrenocorticism)
Intracranial infectious disease (*Neospora caninum,* cerebellar hypoplasia secondary to intrauterine panleukopenia infection)
Intracranial disease (fibrinoid leukodystrophy, neuraxonal dystrophy, Labrador Retriever axonopathy, spongiform encephalopathy, neuronal abiotrophies, subacute necrotizing encephalopathy, lysosomal storage diseases)
Hind end tremor (intervertebral disk herniation, tumors, diskospondylitis, nerve root compression, peripheral neuropathies)
Corticoid-responsive tremor syndrome (formerly "white shaker disease")
Hypomyelination
Spongy degeneration
Tremorgenic toxins (mycotoxins penitrem A and roquefortine produced by *Penicillium* spp. growing on spoiled foods; metaldehyde, hexachlorophene, bromethalin, organophosphates, carbamates, pyrethroids, xanthines, macadamia nuts, strychnine)
Idiopathic head tremor in Doberman Pinschers and Bulldogs
Idiopathic tremor of hindlegs of geriatric dogs

Urine, Discolored

RED, PINK, RED-BROWN, RED-ORANGE, OR ORANGE
Hematuria
Hemoglobinuria
Myoglobinuria
Porphyrinuria
Pyuria

ORANGE-YELLOW
Highly concentrated urine
Urobilin
Bilirubin

YELLOW-BROWN OR GREEN-BROWN
Bile pigments

BROWN TO BLACK
Melanin
Methemoglobin
Myoglobin
Bile pigments

BROWN
Methemoglobin
Melanin

COLORLESS
Dilute urine

MILKY WHITE
Lipid
Pyuria
Crystals

Urticaria/Angioedema

IMMEDIATE HYPERSENSITIVITY REACTION
Insect bites/stings
Food
Drugs/vaccines
Airborne allergens (atopy)

NONIMMUNOLOGIC STIMULUS BY IRRITANT
Weeds
Insects
Physical stimuli (cold, heat, sunlight)
Psychogenic stimuli

Vision Loss, Sudden

See **Blindness.**

Vomiting

GASTRIC DISEASE
  Gastritis
  Parasites
  Foreign body
  Obstruction
  Ulceration
  Neoplasia
  Dilatation/volvulus
  Helicobacter infection
  Gastric ulcer
  Hiatal hernia
  Motility disorders
  Pyloric stenosis
  Gastric antral mucosal hypertrophy

SMALL INTESTINAL DISEASE
  Parasites
  Inflammatory bowel disease
  Foreign body
  Bacterial overgrowth/enteritis
  Hemorrhagic gastroenteritis
  Neoplasia
  Viral enteritis (parvovirus, canine distemper virus)
  Intussusception
  Nonneoplastic infiltrative disease (e.g., pythiosis)

LARGE INTESTINAL DISEASE
  Colitis
  Obstipation
  Parasites

DIETARY
  Indiscretion
  Intolerance
  Allergy
  Pancreatitis

DRUGS
  Cancer chemotherapeutic agents
  Antibiotics (especially erythromycin, tetracycline)
  Nonsteroidal antiinflammatory drugs (NSAIDs)
  Cardiac glycosides
  Apomorphine
  Xylazine
  Penicillamine

EXTRAALIMENTARY TRACT DISEASE
   Peritonitis
   Hepatobiliary disease
   Neoplasia
   Uremia
   Diabetes mellitus/ketoacidosis
   Hyperthyroidism
   Hypoadrenocorticism
   Hepatic disease
   Hepatic encephalopathy
   Septicemia/endotoxemia
   Pyometra
   Acid-base disorders
   Electrolyte disorders
   Hypertriglyceridemia
   Gastrinoma (Zollinger-Ellison syndrome)
   Mastocytosis

INTOXICANTS
Numerous inorganic, organic, and plant toxins can cause gastrointestinal irritation and vomiting.

NEUROLOGIC DISEASE
   Epilepsy, tumor, meningitis, increased intracranial pressure, dysautonomia

Weakness

Very nonspecific clinical sign of disease
   Metabolic disease
   Inflammation
   • Infectious disease (bacterial, viral, fungal, rickettsial, protozoal, parasitic)
   • Immune-mediated disease
   Electrolyte disorders
   • Hypokalemia, hyperkalemia, hyponatremia, hypernatremia, hypocalcemia, hypomagnesemia
   Acid-base disorders
   Anemia
   Endocrine disease
   • Diabetes mellitus, hypothyroidism, hypoadrenocorticism, hyperadrenocorticism, hypoglycemia, hyperparathyroidism, hypoparathyroidism, pheochromocytoma

Cardiovascular disease
Hypotension, hypertension
Respiratory disease
Neuromuscular disease
- Brain disease (encephalitis, cerebrovascular accidents, space-occupying lesions, vestibular disease, idiopathic epilepsy)
- Spinal cord diseases
- Neuropathies (e.g., polyradiculoneuritis, myasthenia gravis, developmental disorders, toxoplasmosis, neosporosis)

Neoplasia
Physical and psychologic stress
Malnutrition
Drugs
- Anticonvulsants, antihistamines, glucocorticoids, tranquilizers, narcotics, cardiac drugs

Pain

Weight Gain

See **Obesity**.

Weight Loss

See **Cachexia and Muscle Wasting**.

Systemic Approach to Differential Diagnosis

Cardiopulmonary Disorders

Arrhythmias
Arterial Thromboembolism
Atrioventricular Valve Disease, Chronic (Mitral or Tricuspid Valve)
Bradycardia, Sinus
Cardiomegaly
Chylothorax
Congenital Heart Disease
Heart Failure
Heartworm Disease
Hypertension
Laryngeal and Pharyngeal Disease
Lower Respiratory Tract Disease
Mediastinal Disease
Myocardial Diseases
Murmurs
Pericardial Effusion
Pleural Effusion
Pulmonary Disease
Pulmonary Edema
Pulmonary Thromboembolism
Tachycardia, Sinus

Arrhythmias

DIFFERENTIAL DIAGNOSIS
    Slow, Irregular Rhythms
        Sinus bradyarrhythmias
        Sinus arrest
        Sick sinus syndrome
        High-grade second-degree atrioventricular (AV) block

    Slow, Regular Rhythms
        Sinus bradycardia
        Complete AV block with ventricular escape rhythm
        Atrial standstill with ventricular escape rhythm

Fast, Irregular Rhythms
Atrial or supraventricular premature contractions
Paroxysmal atrial or supraventricular tachycardia
Atrial flutter
Atrial fibrillation
Ventricular premature contractions
Paroxysmal ventricular tachycardia

Fast, Regular Rhythms
Sinus tachycardia
Sustained supraventricular tachycardia
Sustained ventricular tachycardia

Normal, Irregular Rhythms (require no treatment)
Respiratory sinus arrhythmia
Wandering pacemaker

Arterial Thromboembolism

CLINICAL FINDINGS, CATS
Acute Limb Paresis
Posterior paresis ("saddle" thrombus: most common
    presentation)
Monoparesis
Intermittent claudication
Severe limb pain
Cool distal limbs
Cyanotic nail beds
Arterial pulse absent
Contracture of affected muscles
Vocalization (pain, distress)

Signs of Heart Failure
Systolic murmur
Gallop rhythm
Tachypnea/dyspnea
Weakness/lethargy
Anorexia
Arrhythmias
Hypothermia
Cardiomegaly
Effusions
Pulmonary edema

Hematologic and Biochemical Abnormalities
Azotemia
Increased alanine aminotransferase activity
Increase aspartate aminotransferase activity
Increased lactate dehydrogenase activity
Increased creatine kinase activity
Hyperglycemia
Lymphopenia
Disseminated intravascular coagulation

Atrioventricular Valve Disease, Chronic (Mitral or Tricuspid Valve)

POTENTIAL COMPLICATIONS
Acute Worsening of Pulmonary Edema
Arrhythmias
- Frequent atrial premature contractions
- Paroxysmal atrial/supraventricular contractions
- Atrial fibrillation
- Ventricular tachyarrhythmias

Ruptured chordae tendineae
Iatrogenic volume overload
- Excessive fluid or blood administration
- High-sodium fluids

High sodium intake
Increased cardiac workload
- Physical exertion
- Anemia
- Infection/sepsis
- Hypertension
- Disease of other organ systems (pulmonary, hepatic, renal, endocrine)
- Environmental stress (heat, humidity, cold, etc.)

Inadequate medication for stage of disease
Erratic or improper drug administration
Myocardial degeneration and poor contractility

Causes of Reduced Cardiac Output
Arrhythmias
Ruptured chordae tendineae
Cough related syncope
Left atrial tear, intrapericardial bleeding, cardiac tamponade

Secondary right-sided heart failure
Myocardial degeneration, poor contractility

Bradycardia, Sinus

CAUSES
Normal variation (fit animal)
Hypothyroidism
Hypothermia
Drugs (tranquilizers, anesthetic, β-blockers, calcium entry
  blockers, digitalis)
Increased intracranial pressure
Brain stem lesion
Severe metabolic disease (e.g., uremia)
Ocular pressure
Carotid sinus pressure
High vagal tone
Sinus node disease

Cardiomegaly

DIFFERENTIAL DIAGNOSIS
Generalized Cardiomegaly
Dilated cardiomyopathy
Pericardial effusion
Mitral and tricuspid valve insufficiency
Tricuspid dysplasia
Pericardioperitoneal diaphragmatic hernia
Ventricular septal defect
Patent ductus arteriosus

Left Atrial Enlargement
Mitral valve insufficiency
Hypertrophic cardiomyopathy
Early dilated cardiomyopathy (especially in Doberman
  pinschers)
Subaortic or aortic stenosis

Left Atrial and Ventricular Enlargement
Dilated cardiomyopathy
Hypertrophic cardiomyopathy
Mitral valve insufficiency

Aortic valve insufficiency
Ventricular septal defect
Patent ductus arteriosus
Subaortic or aortic stenosis

Right Atrial and Ventricular Enlargement

Advanced heartworm disease
Chronic severe pulmonary disease
Tricuspid valve insufficiency
Atrial septal defect
Pulmonic stenosis
Tetralogy of Fallot
Reversed-shunting congenital defects
Pulmonary hypertension

Chylothorax

DIAGNOSTIC CRITERIA

Protein concentration is greater than 2.5 g/dL.
Nucleated cell count ranges from 400 to 10,000 /μL.
Predominant cell type on cytology is the small lymphocyte (also see neutrophils, macrophages, plasma cells, and mesothelial cells).
Triglyceride concentration of pleural fluid is greater than that of serum (definitive test).

Congenital Heart Disease

BREED PREDISPOSITIONS

Patent Ductus Arteriosus

Maltese, Pomeranian, Shetland Sheepdog, English Cocker Spaniel, Keeshond, Bichon Frise, toy and miniature Poodle, Yorkshire Terrier, Collie, Cocker Spaniel, German Shepherd, Chihuahua, Kerry Blue Terrier, Labrador Retriever, Newfoundland; female affected more than male

Subaortic Stenosis

Newfoundland, Golden Retriever, Rottweiler, Boxer, German Shepherd, English Bulldog, Great Dane, German Shorthaired Pointer, Bouvier des Flandres, Samoyed

Pulmonic Stenosis
English Bulldog (male>female), Mastiff, Samoyed, Miniature Schnauzer, West Highland White Terrier, Cocker Spaniel, Beagle, Airedale Terrier, Boykin Spaniel, Chihuahua, Scottish Terrier, Boxer, Fox Terrier

Atrial Septal Defect
Samoyed, Doberman Pinscher, Boxer

Ventricular Septal Defect
English Bulldog, English Springer Spaniel, Keeshond, cats

Tricuspid dysplasia
Labrador Retriever, German Shepherd, Boxer, Weimaraner, Great Dane, Old English Sheepdog, Golden Retriever, various other large breeds

Mitral Dysplasia
Bull Terrier, German Shepherd, Great Dane, Golden Retriever, Newfoundland, Mastiff, Rottweiler, cats

Tetralogy of Fallot
Keeshond, English Bulldog

Persistent Right Aortic Arch
German Shepherd, Great Dane, Irish Setter

Cor Triatriatum
Medium- to large-breed dogs, rarely small-breed dogs or cats

Heart Failure

CAUSES OF CHRONIC HEART FAILURE
  Left-Sided Heart Failure
    Volume-Flow Overload
      Mitral endocardiosis
      Mitral/aortic endocardiosis
      Ventricular septal defect
      Patent ductus arteriosis
      Mitral dysplasia

    Myocardial Failure
      Myocardial effusion/infarction
      Drug toxicity (e.g., doxorubicin)

Pressure Overload
Aortic/subaortic stenosis
Systemic hypertension

Restriction of Ventricular Filling
Hypertrophic cardiomyopathy
Restrictive cardiomyopathy

Left- or Right-Sided Heart Failure
Myocardial Failure
Idiopathic dilated cardiomyopathy
Infective myocarditis

Volume-Flow Overload
Chronic anemia
Thyrotoxicosis

Right-Sided Heart Failure
Volume-Flow Overload
Tricuspid endocarditis
Tricuspid endocardiosis
Tricuspid dysplasia

Pressure Overload
Pulmonic stenosis
Heartworm disease
Pulmonary hypertension

Restriction to Ventricular Filling
Cardiac tamponade
Constrictive pericardial disease

SEVERITY
Classification Systems
New York Heart Association Functional Classification
Class I: Heart disease present, but no evidence of heart failure or exercise intolerance; cardiomegaly minimal to absent

Class II: Signs of heart disease with evidence of exercise intolerance; radiographic cardiomegaly present

Class III: Signs of heart failure with normal activity or signs at night (e.g., cough, orthopnea); radiographic signs of significant cardiomegaly and pulmonary edema or pleural/abdominal effusion

Class IV: Severe heart failure with clinical signs at rest or with minimal activity; marked radiographic signs of congestive heart failure (CHF) and cardiomegaly

Forrester's Classification
  Class I: Normal cardiac output and pulmonary
    venous pressure
  Class II: Pulmonary congestion but normal cardiac
    output
  Class III: Low cardiac output and peripheral
    hypoperfusion with no pulmonary congestion
  Class IV: Low cardiac output with pulmonary
    congestion

CLINICAL FINDINGS
Low-Output Signs
Exercise intolerance
Syncope
Weak arterial pulses
Tachycardia
Arrhythmias
Cold extremities

Signs Related to Poor Skeletal Muscle Function
Weight loss
Exercise intolerance
Dyspnea
Decreased muscle mass

Signs Related to Fluid Retention
Left-Sided Heart Failure (Pulmonary Edema)
Dyspnea/orthopnea
Exercise intolerance
Wet lung sounds
Tachypnea
Gallop rhythm
Functional mitral regurgitation
Cyanosis
Cough

Right-Sided Heart Failure
Ascites
Subcutaneous edema
Jugular distension/pulsation
Hepatomegaly
Splenomegaly
Hepatojugular reflux
Gallop rhythm

Bilateral Signs
Pleural effusion (dyspnea, muffled heart sounds,
cough)

Heartworm Disease

CLINICAL FINDINGS
Historical Findings
Asymptomatic
Cough
Dyspnea
Weight loss
Lethargy
Exercise intolerance
Poor condition
Syncope
Abdominal distension

Physical Findings
Weight loss
Right-sided murmur (tricuspid insufficiency)
Split second heart sound
Gallop rhythm
Cough
Pulmonary crackles
Dyspnea
Muffled breath sounds
Cyanosis
Right-sided heart failure
- Jugular distension/pulsation
- Hepatosplenomegaly
- Ascites
Pulmonary thromboembolism
- Dyspnea/tachypnea
- Fever
- Hemoptysis
Cardiac arrhythmias/conduction disturbances (rare)
Caval syndrome
- Hemoglobinuria
- Anemia
- Disseminated intravascular coagulation (DIC)
- Icterus
- Collapse/death

Clinicopathologic Findings
Eosinophilia
Nonregenerative anemia
Neutrophilia
Basophilia

Proteinuria
Hyperbilirubinemia
Azotemia
Thrombocytopenia

Radiographic Signs
Right ventricular enlargement
Prominent main pulmonary artery segment
Increased pulmonary artery size
Tortuous pulmonary vessels
Caudal vena cava enlargement
Hepatosplenomegaly
Ascites
Pleural effusion
Bronchial/interstitial lung disease

Hypertension

PULMONARY HYPERTENSION
Potential Clinical Signs
Ascites
Jugular venous distension/pulsation
Subcutaneous edema
Cachexia
Nonspecific respiratory signs
- Coughing
- Tachypnea
- Respiratory distress
- Increased bronchovesicular sounds
Cyanosis
- Right-to-left cardiac shunts
- Severe respiratory disease
Split or loud pulmonic component to second heart
    sound
Right or left apical systolic murmurs (tricuspid or mitral
    regurgitation)

Radiographic Signs
Cardiomegaly
Right ventricular enlargement
Dilated central pulmonary arteries with tapering toward
    periphery
Eisenmenger's complex (pulmonary undercirculation and
    right-sided heart enlargement)

Left atrial enlargement and perihilar to caudodorsal pulmonary infiltrates (left-sided congestive heart failure)

Echocardiographic Signs

Right ventricular concentric hypertrophy and dilation
Main pulmonary artery and main branch dilation
Systolic flattening of interventricular septum
Paradoxical septal motion
Reduced left ventricular dimensions in severe pulmonary hypertension caused by ventricular underfilling

Laboratory Values

Acidosis
Rule out heartworm disease

SYSTEMIC HYPERTENSION

Diseases and Clinical Findings

Dogs

Renal failure (chronic or acute)
Hyperadrenocorticism
Diabetes mellitus
Pheochromocytoma
Ocular findings
- Hypertensive choroidopathy
- Hypertensive retinopathy
- Intraocular hemorrhage
Neurologic signs not explained by other causes
Left ventricular hypertrophy

Cats

Renal failure (acute or chronic)
Hyperthyroidism
Diabetes mellitus
Ocular findings
- Hypertensive choroidopathy
- Hypertensive retinopathy
- Intraocular hemorrhage
Cardiac signs
- Murmurs
- Gallop rhythm
Neurologic signs

Laryngeal and Pharyngeal Disease

DIFFERENTIAL DIAGNOSIS
Laryngeal paralysis
Brachycephalic airway syndrome
Acute laryngitis
Laryngeal neoplasia
Nasopharyngeal polyp
Abscess
Obstructive laryngitis
Laryngeal collapse
Trauma
Foreign body
Extraluminal mass
Elongated soft palate
Pharyngeal neoplasia
Granuloma
Web formation

CAUSES OF LARYNGEAL PARALYSIS
Idiopathic
Polyneuropathy and Polymyopathy
Idiopathic
Immune-mediated
Endocrinopathy
- Hypothyroidism
- Hypoadrenocorticism

Toxicity
Congenital disease

Ventral Cervical Lesion
Nerve trauma
- Direct trauma
- Inflammation
- Fibrosis

Neoplasia
Other inflammatory or mass lesion

Anterior Thoracic Lesion
Neoplasia
Trauma
- Postoperative
- Other

Other inflammatory or mass lesion

Lower Respiratory Tract Disease

DIFFERENTIAL DIAGNOSIS
Disorders of Trachea and Bronchi
Canine infectious tracheobronchitis
Collapsing trachea
Neoplasia
Allergic bronchitis
Feline bronchitis
Bronchial compression
- Left atrial enlargement
- Hilar lymphadenopathy

Canine chronic bronchitis/bronchiectasis
Parasites *(Oslerus osleri, Filaroides osleri)*
Tracheal tear
Primary ciliary dyskinesia
Airway foreign body

Disorders of Pulmonary Parenchyma
Infectious disease
- Viral pneumonia (canine distemper virus, canine adenovirus, canine parainfluenza, feline calicivirus, feline infectious peritonitis, pneumonia secondary to feline leukemia virus or feline immunodeficiency virus)
- Bacterial pneumonia
- Protozoal pneumonia (toxoplasmosis)
- Fungal pneumonia (blastomycosis, histoplasmosis, coccidioidomycosis)
- Rickettsial disease *(Rickettsia rickettsii, Ehrlichia spp.)*
- Parasitism
  - Heartworm disease
  - Pulmonary parasites (*Paragonimus, Aelurostrongylus, Capillaria, Crenosoma* spp.)

Pulmonary infiltrates with eosinophils
Aspiration pneumonia
Pulmonary neoplasia (primary, metastatic, lymphosarcoma, lymphomatoid granulomatosis, malignant histiocytosis)
Pulmonary contusions
Pulmonary thromboembolism
Pulmonary edema
Acute respiratory distress syndrome
Lung lobe torsion
Pulmonary fibrosis
Pickwickian syndrome (obesity)

Mediastinal Disease

DIFFERENTIAL DIAGNOSIS
  Pneumomediastinum
  Mediastinitis (*Histoplasma, Cryptococcus, Actinomyces, Nocardia, Spirocerca* spp.)
  Mediastinal hemorrhage
  Mediastinal cysts
  Nonneoplastic mediastinal masses (fungal pyogranulomas, abscesses, lymphadenopathy, hematomas)
  Mediastinal neoplasia (lymphosarcoma)
  Thymoma
  Thymic hemorrhage

Myocardial Diseases

DIFFERENTIAL DIAGNOSIS, DOGS
  Dilated Cardiomyopathy
    Primary (idiopathic, most common)
      Genetic (Doberman Pinscher, Boxer, Cocker Spaniel, Great Dane, Portuguese Water Dog)

    Secondary
      Nutritional Deficiencies
        L-Carnitine (Boxer, Doberman Pinscher, Great Dane, Irish Wolfhound, Newfoundland, Cocker Spaniel)
        Taurine

      Myocardial Infection
        Viral myocarditis (acute viral infections, e.g. parvovirus)
        Bacterial myocarditis (secondary to bacteremia from infections elsewhere in body)
        Lyme disease: *Borrelia burgdorferi*
        Protozoal myocarditis (*Trypanosoma cruzi* [Chagas' disease], *Toxoplasma gondii, Neospora caninum, Babesia canis, Hepatozoon canis*)
        Fungal myocarditis (rare, *Aspergillus, Cryptococcus, Coccidioides, Histoplasma, Paecilomyces* spp.)
        Rickettsial myocarditis (rare, *Rickettsia rickettsii, Ehrlichia canis, Bartonella* spp.)
        Algae-like organisms (rare, *Prototheca* spp.)
        Nematode larval migration (*Toxocara* spp.)

Trauma

Ischemia

Infiltrative Neoplasia

Hyperthermia

Irradiation

Electric Shock

Cardiotoxins
Doxorubicin; ethyl alcohol; plant toxins such as
foxglove, black locust, buttercup, lily of the
valley, and gossypol; cocaine; anesthetic
drugs; catecholamines; monensin

Hypertrophic Cardiomyopathy (uncommon in dogs)

Arrhythmogenic Right Ventricular Cardiomyopathy (rare)

Noninfective Myocarditis
Catecholamines, heavy metals, antineoplastic drugs
(doxorubicin, cyclophosphamide, 5-fluorouracil,
interleukin-2, interferon-α), stimulant drugs (thyroid
hormone, cocaine, amphetamines, lithium)
Immune-mediated diseases, pheochromocytoma
Wasp and scorpion stings, snake venom, spider bite

DIFFERENTIAL DIAGNOSIS, CATS
Hypertrophic Cardiomyopathy
Primary (Idiopathic)
Maine coon, Persian, Ragdoll, and American shorthair
may be predisposed.

Secondary
Hyperthyroidism
Hypersomatotropism (acromegaly)
Infiltrative myocardial disease (lymphoma)

Restrictive Cardiomyopathy

Dilated Cardiomyopathy
Taurine-deficient diets
Doxorubicin
End stage of other myocardial metabolic, toxic, or
infectious process

Arrhythmogenic Right Ventricular Cardiomyopathy

Myocarditis
Viral (coronavirus, other viruses)
Bacterial (bacteremia, *Bartonella* spp.)
Protozoal (*Toxoplasma gondii*)

Murmurs

CLINICAL FINDINGS
Systolic Murmurs
Functional murmurs (point of maximal impulse [PMI] over left-sided heart base, decrescendo or crescendo-decrescendo)
- Innocent puppy murmurs
- Physiologic murmurs (anemia, fever, high sympathetic tone, hyperthyroidism, peripheral arteriovenous fistula, hypoproteinemia, athletic heart)

Mitral valve insufficiency (left apex, typically holosystolic)
Ejection murmurs (typically left-sided heart base)
- Subaortic stenosis (low left base and right base)
- Pulmonic stenosis (high left base)
- Dynamic muscular obstruction

Right-sided murmurs (usually holosystolic)
- Tricuspid insufficiency (right apex, may see jugular pulse)
- Ventricular septal defect (PMI over right sternal border)

Diastolic Murmurs
Aortic insufficiency from bacterial endocarditis (left-sided heart base)
Aortic valve congenital malformations (left base)
Aortic valve degenerative disease (left base)
Pulmonic insufficiency (left base)

Continuous Murmurs
Patent ductus arteriosus (PMI high left base above pulmonic area)

Concurrent Systolic and Diastolic Murmurs (To-and-Fro Murmurs)
Subaortic stenosis with aortic insufficiency
Pulmonic stenosis with pulmonic insufficiency

GRADING

Grade I: Very soft murmur; heard only in quiet surroundings after minutes of listening

Grade II: Soft murmur but easily heard

Grade III: Moderate-intensity murmur

Grade IV: Loud murmur; no precordial thrill

Grade V: Loud murmur with palpable precordial thrill

Grade VI: Very loud murmur; can be heard with stethoscope off chest wall; palpable precordial thrill

Pericardial Effusion

DIFFERENTIAL DIAGNOSIS

Bacterial Pericarditis

Secondary to foxtail (*Hordeum* spp.) migration

Secondary to penetrating animal bite

Disseminated tuberculosis

Fungal Pericarditis

Coccidioidomysosis

Aspergillosis

Actinomycosis

Viral Pericarditis

Feline infectious peritonitis (FIP)

Canine distemper virus

Protozoal Pericarditis

Toxoplasmosis

Other systemic protozoal infections

Left Atrial Rupture (Secondary to Mitral Valve Disease)

Neoplasia

Hemangiosarcoma

Mesothelioma

Heart base tumor (aortic body tumor or chemodectoma, ectopic thyroid tumor, ectopic parathyroid tumor, connective tissue neoplasms)

Lymphosarcoma

Rhabdomyosarcoma

Other

Penetrating trauma

Pericardioperitoneal diaphragmatic hernia

Hypoalbuminemia
Pericardial cyst
Coagulation disorders
Congestive heart failure
Uremia
Idiopathic

Pleural Effusion

DIFFERENTIAL DIAGNOSIS
Transudates and Modified Transudates
Right-sided heart failure
Pericardial disease
Hypoalbuminemia
Neoplasia
Diaphragmatic hernia

Nonseptic Exudates
Feline infectious peritonitis (FIP)
Neoplasia
Diaphragmatic hernia
Lung lobe torsion

Septic Exudates
Pyothorax

Chylous Effusion
Chylothorax

Hemorrhage
Trauma
Bleeding disorder
Neoplasia
Lung lobe torsion

Pulmonary Disease

DIFFERENTIAL DIAGNOSIS BASED ON RADIOGRAPHIC
PATTERNS
Alveolar Pattern
Pulmonary edema
Bacterial pneumonia
Aspiration pneumonia

Hemorrhage
- Neoplasia
- Fungal pneumonia (severe)
- Pulmonary contusion
- Thromboembolic disease
- Systemic coagulopathy

Bronchial Pattern
Feline bronchitis
Allergic bronchitis
Bacterial bronchitis
Canine chronic bronchitis
Bronchiectasis
Pulmonary parasites

Vascular Pattern
Enlarged Arteries
Heartworm disease
Thromboembolic disease
Pulmonary hypertension

Enlarged Veins
Left-sided heart failure

Enlarged Artieries and Veins (Pulmonary Overcirculation)

Left-to-Right Shunts
Patent ductus arteriosus
Ventricular septal defect
Atrial septal defect

Small Arteries and Veins
Pulmonary Undercirculation
Cardiovascular shock
Hypovolemia
- Severe dehydration
- Blood loss
- Hypoadrenocorticism
Pulmonic valve stenosis

Hyperinflation of Lungs
Feline bronchitis
Allergic bronchitis

Nodular Interstitial Pattern
Mycotic infection
- Blastomycosis

- Histoplasmosis
- Coccidioidomycosis

Neoplasia

Pulmonary parasites
- *Aelurostrongylus* infection
- *Paragonimus* infection

Pulmonary abscess
- Bacterial pneumonia
- Foreign body

Pulmonary infiltrates with eosinophils

Miscellaneous inflammatory diseases

Inactive lesions

Reticular Interstitial Patterns

Infection
- Viral pneumonia
- Bacterial pneumonia
- Toxoplasmosis
- Mycotic pneumonia

Parasitic infestation

Neoplasia

Pulmonary fibrosis

Pulmonary infiltrates with eosinophils

Miscellaneous inflammatory diseases

Hemorrhage (mild)

Pulmonary Edema

CAUSES

Vascular Overload

Cardiogenic
- Left-sided heart murmur
- Left-to-right shunt

Overhydration

Decreased Plasma Oncotic Pressure

Hypoalbuminemia
- Gastrointestinal loss
- Renal loss (glomerular disease)
- Liver disease (lack of production)
- Iatrogenic overhydration

Increased Vascular Permeability

Sepsis

Drugs or toxins

    Snake toxins
    Cisplatin (cats)
    Trauma
- Pulmonary
- Multisystemic

    Inhaled toxins
- Smoke inhalation
- Gastric acid aspiration
- Oxygen toxicity

    Electrocution
    Pancreatitis
    Uremia
    Disseminated intravascular coagulation
    Inflammation

Other Causes
    Thromboembolism
    Upper airway obstruction
    Near-drowning
    Neurogenic edema
- Seizures
- Head trauma

Lymphatic Obstruction (rare)
    Neoplasia

Pulmonary Thromboembolism

CAUSES
Embolization of Thrombi
    Heartworm disease
- Venous stasis
- Endothelial injury
- Hypercoagulability

    Immune-mediated hemolytic anemia
    Neoplasia
    Cardiac disease
    Protein-losing nephropathy
    Protein-losing enteropathy
    Hyperadrenocorticism
    Disseminated intravascular coagulation
    Sepsis
    Trauma
    Recent surgery

Embolization of parasites
Heartworm disease

Embolization of Fat

Embolization of Neoplastic Cells

Tachycardia, Sinus

CAUSES
Anxiety/fear
Excitement
Exercise
Pain
Hyperthyroidism
Hyperthermia/fever
Anemia
Hypoxia
Shock
Hypotension
Sepsis
Drugs (anticholinergics, sympathomimetics)
Toxicity (e.g., chocolate, hexachlorophene)
Electric shock

Section II

Dermatologic Disorders

Allergic Skin Disease

CLINICAL FINDINGS

Flea Allergy

Dogs
Papular rash
Caudal distribution of lesions most common

Cats
Miliary dermatitis, especially over caudal back, around neck and chin
Eosinophilic granuloma complex

Atopy and Cutaneous Signs of Food Hypersensitivity
Signs of these two types of allergy are very similar.
Atopy tends to occur primarily in young adults, whereas food hypersensitivity can begin at any age. Atopy is usually seasonal at first, but may become less seasonal.

Dogs
Papular rash
Pruritus and self-trauma
Lesions of face, ears, feet, and perineum
Recurrent otitis externa
Excoriation
Lichenification
Pigmentary changes
Secondary pyoderma

Cats
Miliary dermatitis
Eosinophilic dermatitis

Allergic Contact Dermatitis
Rarest of allergic dermatoses
Lesions tend to be confined to hairless or sparsely haired skin (ventral abdomen, neck, and chest; ventral paws but not pads; perineum; lateral aspect of pinnae).
Acutely: Erythema, macules, papules, vesicles
Chronically: Alopecic plaques, hyperpigmentation, hypopigmentation, excoriation, lichenification

Alopecia, Endocrine

CAUSES
Hypothyroidism
Hyperadrenocorticism
Diabetes mellitus
Adrenal sex hormone deficiency
Growth hormone deficiency (pituitary dwarfism)
Growth hormone-responsive dermatosis in adult dogs
Castration-responsive dermatosis
Hyperestrogenism
- Sertoli cell tumor (male dog)
- Intact female dog

Hypoestrogenism (poorly understood)
- Estrogen-responsive dermatosis of spayed female dogs
- Feline endocrine alopecia

Hypoadrogenism
- Testosterone-responsive dermatosis (male dog)
- Feline endocrine alopecia

Telogen defluxion (effluvium): often after recent pregnancy or diestrus
Progestin excess (excess of progesterone or 17-hydroxyprogesterone)

CLINICAL FINDINGS
Nonspecific Features of Endocrine Disease
Bilaterally symmetric alopecia
Follicular dilation, follicular keratosis, follicular atrophy
Orthokeratotic hyperkeratosis
Predominance of telogen hair follicles
Sebaceous gland atrophy

Epidermal atrophy
Thin dermis
Epidermal melanosis
Dermal collagen atrophy

Features Suggestive of Specific Endocrine Disorder
Hypothyroidism
- Vacuolated and/or hypertrophied arrector pili muscles, increased dermal mucin content, thick dermis

Hyperadrenocorticism
- Calcinosis cutis, comedones, absence of erector pili muscles

Hyposomatotropism
- Decreased amount and size of dermal elastin fibers

Growth hormone and castration-responsive dermatoses
- Excessive trichilemmal keratinization (flame follicles)

Erosions and Ulcerations of Skin or Mucous Membranes

DIFFERENTIAL DIAGNOSIS, DOGS
Excoriation from Any Pruritic Skin Disease

Infection
Bacterial Pyoderma
Surface (pyotraumatic moist dermatitis, intertrigo)
Deep (folliculitis, furunculosis, bacterial stomatitis)

Fungal
Yeast infection (*Malassezia pachydermatis, Candida* spp.)
Dermatophytosis
Systemic fungal infection (blastomycosis, coccidioidomycosis, cryptococcosis, histoplasmosis, others)
Subcutaneous mycoses (pythiosis, zygomycosis, phaeohyphomycosis, sporotrichosis, eumycotic mycetoma, others)

Parasitic
Demodicosis

Neoplasia
Squamous cell carcinoma
Epitheliotrophic lymphoma

Metabolic Derangements
Uremia/renal failure
Necrolytic migratory erythema
Calcinosis cutis (hyperadrenocorticism)

Physical/Chemical Injury
Drug reactions
Urine scald
Thermal injury (burn, freeze)
Solar injury

Immune-Mediated Disorders
Discoid lupus erythematosus (DLE)
Pemphigus
Uveodermatologic syndrome
Miscellaneous autoimmune subepidermal
vesiculobullous diseases (bullous pemphigoid,
epidermolysis acquisita, linear IgA bullous disease,
mucocutaneous pemphigoid, bullous systemic lupus
type 1)

Miscellaneous
Arthropod bites
Dermatomyositis
Dystrophic epidermolysis bullosa, junctional
epidermolysis bullosa
Idiopathic ulceration of collies
Toxic epidermal necrolysis, erythema multiforme

DIFFERENTIAL DIAGNOSIS, CATS
Infection
Viral
Calicivirus
Herpesvirus

Bacterial
Atypical mycobacteriosis

Fungal
Cryptococcosis
Systemic and subcutaneous mycoses
Sporotrichosis

Neoplasia
Squamous cell carcinomas (especially white,
outdoor cats)
Fibrosarcoma
Cutaneous lymphoma

Metabolic Derangements
Uremia/renal disease

Physical/Chemical Injury
Thermal
Drug reactions

Immune-Mediated Disorders
Bullous pemphigoid
Pemphigus foliaceus
Plasma cell pododermatitis
Toxic epidermal necrolysis

Inflammatory/Allergic Disorders
Eosinophilic plaque
Indolent ulcer
Arthropod bites

Miscellaneous/Idiopathic
Dystrophic epidermolysis bullosa
Idiopathic ulceration of dorsal neck
Junctional epidermolysis bullosa

Folliculitis

DIFFERENTIAL DIAGNOSIS
Superficial Folliculitis
Inflammation of hair follicles
- Bacterial pyoderma
- Fungal (dermatophytosis)
- Parasitic (demodicosis, *Pelodera* dermatitis)

Deep Folliculitis/Furunculosis
Inflammation of hair follicles with subsequent follicular rupture into dermis and subcutaneous tissues
- Deep pyodermas

Otitis Externa, Chronic

PRIMARY CAUSES
Allergy
Atopy
Adverse reactions to foods
Contact dermatitis

Parasites
Otodectes cynotis
Notoedres cati
Sarcoptes scabiei
Demodex spp.
Chiggers
Flies
Ticks (spinous ear tick)

Dermatophytes

Foreign Bodies
Foxtails, hair, etc.

Glandular Conditions
Ceruminous gland hyperplasia
Sebaceous gland hyperplasia or hypoplasia
Altered type or rate of secretions

Autoimmune Diseases
Systemic lupus erythematosus (SLE)
Pemphigus foliaceus/erythematosus
Cold agglutinin disease

Viruses
Distemper

Miscellaneous
Solar dermatitis
Frostbite
Vasculitis/vasculopathy
Juvenile cellulitis
Eosinophilic dermatitis
Sterile eosinophilic folliculitis
Relapsing polychondritis

PREDISPOSING FACTORS
Conformation
Stenotic canals
Hair in canals
Pendulous pinnae
Hairy, concave pinna

Excessive Moisture
Swimmer's ear
High-humidity climate

Excessive Cerumen Production
Secondary to underlying disease
Primary (idiopathic)

Treatment Effects
Trauma from cotton swabs
Topical irritants
Superinfections from altering microflora

Obstructive Ear Disease
Polyps
Granulomas
Tumors

Systemic Disease
Immunosuppression
Debilitation
Negative catabolic states

PERPETUATING FACTORS
Bacteria

Yeast

Progressive Pathologic Changes
Hyperkeratosis
Hyperplasia
Epithelial folds
Apocrine gland hypertrophy
Hidradenitis
Fibrosis

Otitis Media
Purulent
Caseated or keratinous
Cholesteatoma
Proliferative
Destructive osteomyelitis

Parasitic Dermatoses

CLASSIFICATION
Fleas
Flea infestation
Flea allergy dermatitis
- Caudal distribution of lesions (dogs)
- Miliary dermatitis (cats)

Demodicosis
Follicular infection *(Demodex canis, Demodex felis)*
Epidermal infection (*Demodex gatoi,* short-tailed
demodectic mite of dogs)

Sarcoptic Mange
Sarcoptes scabiei (dogs, rarely cats)
Notoedres cati (cats, rarely dogs)

Ear Mites
Otodectes cynotis (common in both dogs and cats)

Cheyletiellosis
Cheyletiella yasguri (primary host is dogs)
C. blakei (primary host is cats)
C. parasitovorax (primary host is rabbits)
All *Cheyletiella* species freely contagious from one species
to another

Chiggers
Larval stage (six-legged bright red or orange) is the
parasitic stage; nymph and adult are free living.

Ticks
Brown dog tick *(Rhipicephalus sanguineus)*
American dog tick *(Dermacentor variabilis)*
Rocky Mountain wood tick *(Dermacentor andersoni)*
Lone star tick *(Amblyomma americanum)*
Deer tick *(Ixodes dammini)*: primary vector of *Borrelia
burgdorferi*
Spinous ear tick *(Otobius megnini)*

Lice
Sucking lice of dogs *(Linognathus setosus)*
Biting lice of dogs *(Trichodectes canis, Heterodoxus springer)*
Lice of cats *(Felicola subrostrata)*

Insects of Order Diptera
Mosquitoes: eosinophilic dermatitis (especially cats)
Black flies, stable flies, horn flies, houseflies: attack ear
pinnae of dogs
Myiasis (development of fly larvae in skin or haircoat):
screwworm, blow flies, flesh flies

Helminth Parasites
Hookworm dermatitis *(Ancylostoma, Uncinaria)*
Pelodera dermatitis *(Pelodera strongyloides)*
Dracunculiasis *(Dracunculus insignis)*

Pigmentation

DIFFERENTIAL DIAGNOSIS FOR CHANGES IN SKIN PIGMENTATION

Hypopigmentation

Vitiligo (Tervuren, Rottweiler, Doberman Pinscher, Newfoundland, Collie, German Shorthaired Pointer, Old English Sheepdog, Siamese cat)

Uveodermatologic syndrome (northern breeds such as Siberian Husky, Samoyed, Akita)

Acquired idiopathic hypopigmentation of nose (Labrador Retriever, Siberian Husky, Samoyed, Poodle, German Shepherd)

Discoid lupus (German Shepherd, Collie, others)

Dermatomyositis (Collie, Shetland Sheepdog, Beauceron Shepherd)

Hyperpigmentation

Postinflammatory Hyperpigmentation

Any Chronic Pruritic Skin Disease

Atopy

Adverse food reactions

Pyoderma

Malassezia dermatitis

Sarcoptic mange

Many others

Demodicosis

Endocrinopathies

Hypothyroidism

Hyperadrenocortism

Dermatophytosis

Nevus

Neoplasia (melanoma)

Pyoderma

DIFFERENTIAL DIAGNOSIS

Surface Pyoderma

Pyotraumatic dermatitis (acute moist dermatitis, "hot spot")

Intertrigo (skin fold dermatitis)

Superficial Pyoderma

Impetigo (subcorneal pustules of sparsely haired skin)
- Puppy pyoderma

Bullous impetigo
- Hyperadrenocorticism, hypothyroidism, diabetes mellitus

Mucocutaneous pyoderma
- Dogs (German Shepherds predisposed)

Superficial bacterial folliculitis
- *Staphylococcus intermedius* most common
- Local trauma secondary to pruritus (allergy, fleas, scabies, demodicosis, etc.)

Dermatophilosis (rare, actinomycotic superficial crusting dermatitis)

Deep Pyoderma

Always secondary to predisposing problem

Localized lesion (laceration, penetrating wound, animal bite, foreign body)

Generalized (suspect underlying systemic disease)

Clinical syndromes associated with deep pyoderma
- Deep folliculitis, furunculosis, cellulitis
- Pyotraumatic folliculitis
- Muzzle folliculitis and furunculosis
- Pododermatitis (interdigital pyoderma)
- German Shepherd dog folliculitis, furunculosis, cellulitis
- Acral lick furunculosis
- Anaerobic cellulites
- Subcutaneous abscesses
- Bacterial pseudomycetoma
- Mycobacterial granulomas
  - Cutaneous tuberculosis *(Mycobacterium tuberculosis, M. bovis)*
  - Feline leprosy *(M. lepraemurium)*
  - Opportunistic mycobacterial granulomas
- Actinomycosis
- Actinobacillosis
- Nocardiosis

Miscellaneous Bacterial Infections

Brucellosis, plague, borreliosis, trichomycosis axillaris, L-form infections

Endocrinologic and Metabolic Disorders

Acromegaly

In dogs, acromegaly is caused by endogenous progesterone from the luteal phase of the estrous cycle or by exogenous progesterone used for estrous prevention. Elevated progesterone, in turn, stimulates excessive growth hormone secretion of mammary origin. In cats, acromegaly is caused by a pituitary adenoma, usually a macroadenoma, which secretes excessive amounts of growth hormone. Physical changes are less pronounced in cats than in dogs.

CLINICAL FINDINGS, DOGS

Hypertrophy of mouth, tongue, and pharynx
Thick skin folds, myxedema, hypertrichosis
Prognathism
Wide interdental spacing

Visceral organomegaly
Insulin-resistant diabetes mellitus

CLINICAL FINDINGS, CATS
Physical changes most pronounced on head, but all the
physical changes listed for dogs may be seen.
Insulin-resistant diabetes mellitus (severe)
Degenerative arthropathy/lameness
Polyuria/polydipsia
Polyphagia
Panting
Lethargy/exercise intolerance
Dyspnea secondary to hypertrophic cardiomyopathy and
heart failure
Neurologic signs when macroadenoma becomes large
- Lethargy, stupor
- Adipsia
- Anorexia
- Temperature deregulation
- Circling
- Seizures
- Pituitary dysfunction
  - Hypogonadism
  - Hypothyroidism
  - Hypoadrenocorticism

Adrenal Tumors

DIFFERENTIAL DIAGNOSIS
Nonfunctional Adrenal Tumor (dog, rarely cat)
No hormone secreted
Diagnosis by exclusion
Histopathology

Functional Adrenocortical Tumor
Cortisol-Secreting Tumor
Hyperadrenocorticism (Cushing's syndrome) (dog,
rarely cat)
Diagnosis by adrenocorticotropic hormone (ACTH)
stimulation test or low-dose dexamethasone
suppression test

Aldosterone-Secreting Tumor
Hyperaldosteronism (Conn's syndrome) (cat,
rarely dog)

Diagnosis by assessing Na/K, ACTH stimulation test
(measure aldosterone)

Progesterone-Secreting Tumor
Mimics hyperadrenocorticism (cat, less
commonly dog)
Diagnosis by measuring serum progesterone

Steroid Hormone Precursor–Secreting Tumor
17-hydroxyprogesterone
Mimics hyperadrenocorticism (dog)
Diagnosis by ACTH stimulation test (measure steroid
hormone precursors)
Deoxycorticosterone
Mimics hyperadrenocorticism (dog)
Diagnosis by ACTH stimulation test (measure steroid
hormone precursors)

Functional Adrenomedullary Tumor
Epinephrine-Secreting Tumor
Pheochromocytosis (dog, rarely cat)
Diagnosis by exclusion, histopathology

Cretinism (Hypothyroidism in Puppies)

CLINICAL FINDINGS
Dwarfism
Short, broad skull
Enlarged cranium
Shortened limbs
Shortened mandible
Mental dullness
Alopecia
Retention of puppy coat
Kyphosis
Inappetence
Constipation
Gait abnormalities
Delayed dental eruption
Dry coat
Thick skin
Lethargy
Dyspnea
Goiter

Diabetes Insipidus

DIFFERENTIAL DIAGNOSIS
Features of diabetes insipidus include polyuria, polydipsia, and a near-continuous demand for water. Only the following three disorders can cause the degree of polyuria and dilute urine seen with diabetes insipidus:

- Central diabetes insipidus
- Nephrogenic diabetes insipidus
- Primary polydipsia

CAUSES IN DOGS AND CATS

Central Diabetes Insipidus

Idiopathic
Traumatic
Neoplasia
- Craniopharyngioma
- Chromophobe adenoma
- Chromophobe adenocarcinoma
- Metastatic neoplasia

Pituitary malformation
Cysts
Inflammation
Familial?

Nephrogenic Diabetes Insipidus

Polyuria caused by nonresponsiveness to antidiuretic hormone (ADH).

Primary idiopathic
Primary familial (Husky)
Secondary acquired
- Renal insufficiency or failure
- Hyperadrenocorticism
- Hypoadrenocorticism
- Hepatic insufficiency
- Pyometra
- Hypercalcemia
- Hypokalemia
- Postobstructive diuresis
- Diabetes mellitus
- Normoglycemic glucosuria
- Hyperthyroidism
- Iatrogenic or drug induced
- Renal medullary solute washout

Diabetic Ketoacidosis

CLINICAL FINDINGS
No signs may be seen early with diabetic ketoacidosis.

Historical findings
Lethargy
Anorexia
Vomiting

Physical Examination Findings
Dehydration
Depression
Weakness
Tachypnea
Vomiting
Acetone odor on breath
Slow, deep breaths (secondary to metabolic acidosis)
Abdominal pain/abdominal distension secondary to
    concurrent pancreatitis

Clinicopathologic findings
Hyperglycemia
Metabolic acidosis
Hypercholesterolemia/lipemia
Increased alkaline phosphatase (ALP)
Increased alanine aminotransferase (ALT)
Increased blood urea nitrogen (BUN)/creatinine
Hyponatremia
Hypochloremia
Hypokalemia
Increased amylase/lipase
Hyperosmolality
Glycosuria
Ketonuria
Urinary tract infection

Diabetes Mellitus

POTENTIAL FACTORS IN ETIOPATHOGENESIS
Obesity
Pancreatitis
Immune-mediated insulitis
Concurrent hormonal disease

- Hyperadrenocorticism
- Diestrus-induced excess of growth hormone
- Hypothyroidism

Genetics (dog, possibly cat)

Drugs

- Glucocorticoids
- Megestrol acetate (cat)

Infection

Concurrent illness

- Renal insufficiency
- Cardiac disease

Hyperlipidemia (dog, possibly cat)

Islet amyloidosis

CLINICOPATHOLOGIC ABNORMALITIES, UNCOMPLICATED DIABETES MELLITUS

Complete Blood Count

Often normal

Leukocytosis if pancreatitis or infection present

Serum Chemistry

Hyperglycemia

Mild increase in alkaline phosphatase (ALP) and alanine
aminotransferase (ALT)

Hypercholesterolemia/hypertriglyceridemia

Urinalysis

Urine specific gravity normal to mildly decreased
(> 1.025)

Glycosuria

Variable ketonuria

Bacteriuria

Proteinuria

Ancillary Tests

Increased amylase/lipase if pancreatitis present

Normal serum trypsin-like immunoreactivity (TLI)

Low TLI with exocrine pancreatic insufficiency

High TLI with acute pancreatitis

Normal to high TLI with chronic pancreatitis

Low to normal serum insulin with insulin-dependent
diabetes mellitus

Low, normal, or increased serum insulin with
non–insulin-dependent diabetes mellitus

POTENTIAL COMPLICATIONS

Common

Iatrogenic hypoglycemia
Polyuria/polydipsia
Weight loss
Cataracts (dog)
Bacterial infections (especially urinary tract infection)
Ketoacidosis
Pancreatitis
Peripheral neuropathy (cat)
Hepatic lipidosis

Uncommon
Peripheral neuropathy
Glomerulopathy
Glomerulosclerosis
Retinopathy
Exocrine pancreatic insufficiency
Gastric paresis
Diabetic diarrhea
Diabetic dermatopathy

CAUSES OF INSULIN RESISTANCE OR INEFFECTIVENESS IN DOGS AND CATS
Caused by Insulin Therapy
Improper administration
Inadequate dose
Inactive insulin
Diluted insulin
Somogyi effect
Inappropriate insulin administration
Impaired insulin absorption
Antiinsulin antibody excess

Caused by Concurrent Disorder
Obesity
Hyperadrenocorticism
Hypothyroidism (dog)
Hyperthyroidism (cat)
Urinary tract infection
Oral infections
Chronic inflammation/pancreatitis
Diestrus (bitch)
Acromegaly (cat)
Renal insufficiency
Hepatic insufficiency
Cardiac insufficiency
Glucagonoma

Pheochromocytoma
Exocrine pancreatic insufficiency
Hyperlipidemia
Neoplasia

CLINICAL FINDINGS ASSOCIATED WITH INSULIN-SECRETING TUMORS
Seizures
Weakness
Collapse
Ataxia
Polyphagia
Weight gain
Muscle fasciculations
Posterior weakness (neuropathy)
Lethargy
Nervousness
Unusual behavior

Gastrinoma (Zollinger-Ellison Syndrome)

CLINICAL FINDINGS
Clinical Signs
Vomiting
Weight loss
Anorexia
Diarrhea
Gastric and duodenal ulceration
Hematochezia
Melena
Lethargy/depression
Abdominal pain
Esophageal pain and ulceration
Regurgitation
Fever
Polydipsia
Thin body condition
Pallor

Clinicopathologic Findings
Regenerative anemia
Hypoproteinemia
Neutrophilic leukocytosis
Hypoalbuminemia

Hypocalcemia
Mild increases in hepatic enzymes
Hypochloremia
Hypokalemia
Metabolic acidosis
Hyperglycemia, hypoglycemia (uncommon)

Glucagonoma

CLINICAL FINDINGS IN DOGS
Clinical Signs
Necrolytic migratory erythema (crusting skin rash of
elbows, hocks, nose, scrotum, flank, ventral abdomen,
distal extremities, and mucocutaneous junctions of
mouth, eyes, and vulva)
Footpad lesions
Glucose intolerance/diabetes mellitus (caused by excess
glycogenolysis and gluconeogenesis)
Lethargy
Weight loss
Decreased appetite
Muscle atrophy
Peripheral lymphadenopathy

Clinicopathologic Findings
Hyperglycemia
Nonregenerative anemia
Increased hepatic enzymes
Decreased albumin
Decreased globulin
Decreased blood urea nitrogen (BUN)
Decreased cholesterol
Glucosuria
Abdominal ultrasound lesions
- Increased echogenicity of portal and hepatic vein
walls
- Diffuse hyperechogenicity
- Multiple small hypoechoic foci

Hyperadrenocorticism

CLINICAL FINDINGS
  Potential Clinical Signs
    Polyuria/polydipsia
    Alopecia
    Pendulous abdomen
    Hepatomegaly
    Polyphagia
    Muscle weakness
    Muscle atrophy
    Pyoderma
    Comedones
    Panting
    Pacing/restlessness
    Hyperpigmentation
    Systemic hypertension
    Testicular atrophy
    Anestrus
    Calcinosis cutis
    Facial nerve paralysis
    Pulmonary thromboembolism

  Potential Clinicopathologic Findings
    Urinary tract infection/pyelonephritis
    Decreased urine specific gravity
    Increased serum alkaline phosphatase (ALP)
    Increased alanine aminotransferase (ALT)
    Hypercholesterolemia
    Hypertriglyceridemia
    Hyperglycemia (mild to moderate)
    Diabetes mellitus (uncommon)
    Increased serum bile acids
    Decreased BUN and creatinine (secondary to diuresis)
    Hypophosphatemia
    Stress leukogram
      • Neutrophilia
      • Lymphopenia
      • Eosinopenia
      • Monocytosis
    Thrombocytosis
    Decreased total serum thyroxine (T_4) or free T_4
    Urolithiasis

Hyperglycemia

DIFFERENTIAL DIAGNOSIS
Diabetes mellitus
Stress (physiologic in cat)
Hyperadrenocorticism
Drug therapy
- Glucocorticoids
- Progestagens
- Megestrol acetate
- Thiazide diuretics

Dextrose-containing fluids
Parenteral nutrition
Postprandial effect (diets containing monosaccharides, disaccharides, propylene glycol)
Exocrine pancreatic neoplasia
Renal insufficiency
Acromegaly (cat)
Pheochromocytoma (dog)
Diestrus (bitch)
Head trauma

Hypoadrenocorticism

POTENTIAL CLINICAL FINDINGS
   Clinical Signs
      Lethargy/depression
      Episodic weakness
      Vomiting
      Anorexia
      Waxing and waning illness
      Weight loss/failure to gain weight
      Bradycardia
      Dehydration/hypovolemia
      Diarrhea
      Polyuria or polydipsia
      Collapse
      Syncope
      Restlessness/shaking/shivering
      Regurgitation
      Muscle cramping
      Melena
      Abdominal pain

Potential Clinicopathologic Findings
Hyponatremia
Hyperkalemia
Hypochloremia
Decreased sodium/potassium ratio (< 24:1)
Azotemia
- Increased blood urea nitrogen (BUN)
- Increased creatinine
- Increased phosphate
Decreased bicarbonate and total CO_2 concentrations
Hypercalcemia
Hypoglycemia
Hypoalbuminemia
Lymphocytosis
Eosinophilia
Relative neutropenia
Anemia (usually nonregenerative)
Variable urine specific gravity

Hypoglycemia

DIFFERENTIAL DIAGNOSIS

Excess Secretion of Insulin or Insulin-Like Factors
Insulinoma
Extrapancreatic tumor
Islet cell hyperplasia

Decreased Glucose Production
Toy breeds
Neonates
Malnutrition
Pregnancy
Fasting
Hypoadrenocorticism
Hypopituitarism
Growth hormone deficiency
Liver disease (portal caval shunt, chronic
  fibrosis/cirrhosis)
Glycogen storage diseases

Excess Glucose Consumption
Sepsis
Extreme exercise

Drug-Associated Causes
Insulin
Oral hypoglycemics
Many other drugs reported to cause hypoglycemia in
humans

Spurious
Blood cells not promptly separated from serum

Hyponatremia/Hyperkalemia

DIFFERENTIAL DIAGNOSIS
Hypoadrenocorticism

Renal or Urinary Tract Disease
Urethral obstruction
Acute renal failure
Chronic oliguric or anuric renal failure
Postobstructive diuresis
Nephrotic syndrome

Severe Gastrointestinal Disease
Parasitic infestation
  • Whipworm (trichuriasis)
  • Roundworm (ascariasis)
  • Hookworm (ancylostomiasis)
Salmonellosis
Viral enteritis
  • Parvovirus
  • Canine distemper virus
Gastric dilatation/volvulus
Gastrointestinal perforation
Severe malabsorption
Hemorrhagic gastroenteritis
Pancreatic disease

Severe Hepatic Failure
Cirrhosis
Neoplasia

Severe Metabolic or Respiratory Acidosis

Congestive Heart Failure

Massive Release of Potassium into Extracellular Fluid
Crush injury
Aortic thrombosis
Rhabdomyolysis
- Heat stroke
- Exertional

Massive sepsis
Massive hemolysis

Pleural Effusion

Pregnancy

Lymphangiosarcoma

Pseudohyperkalemia
Akitas and related breeds
Severe leukocytosis (> 100,000 /mm^3)
Severe thrombocytosis (> 1 million/mm^3)

Diabetes Mellitus

Primary Polydipsia

Inappropriate Antidiuretic Hormone (ADH) Secretion

Drug Induced
Potassium-sparing diuretics
Nonsteroidal antiinflammatory drugs (NSAIDs)
Angiotensin-converting enzyme (ACE) inhibitors
Potassium-containing fluids

Insulinoma

DIFFERENTIAL DIAGNOSIS FOR INSULIN-SECRETING β-CELL NEOPLASIA

Excess Insulin or Insulin-Like Factors
Insulinoma
Extrapancreatic tumor
Islet cell hyperplasia

Decreased Glucose Production
Hypoadrenocorticism
Hypopituitarism
Growth hormone deficiency
Liver disease

Glycogen storage diseases
Neonates
Toy breeds
Fasting
Malnutrition
Pregnancy

Excess Glucose Consumption
Sepsis
Extreme exercise

Drug-Associated Causes
Insulin
Oral hypoglycemics (sulfonylurea)
Salicylates (e.g., aspirin)
Acetaminophen
β-blockers
$β_2$-agonists
Ethanol
Monoamine oxidase inhibitors
Tricyclic antidepressants
Angiotensin-converting enzyme (ACE) inhibitors
Antibiotics (e.g., tetracycline)
Lidocaine overdose
Lithium

Factitious Hypoglycemia
Failure to separate blood cells from serum promptly
Severe polycythemia or leukocytosis when serum
    separation delayed

Parathyroidism

HYPERPARATHYROIDISM, PRIMARY—CLINICAL FINDINGS
Clinical Signs
Polyuria/polydipsia
Weight loss
Anorexia
Lethargy, listlessness
Urinary tract infection (UTI)
Urolithiasis
Vomiting
Constipation
Mental dullness, obtundation, coma
Weakness, muscle wasting, shivering

Clinicopathologic Findings
Hypercalcemia
Increased ionized calcemia
Low normal to low serum phosphorus
Decreased urine specific gravity
Hematuria
Pyuria
Crystalluria
Bacteriuria

HYPOPARATHYROIDISM—CLINICAL FINDINGS
Clinical Signs
Seizures
Facial rubbing
Splinted abdomen
Stiff gait
Muscle fasciculations
Fever
Paroxysmal tachyarrhythmias
Muffled heart sounds
Weak pulses
Disorientation

Clinicopathologic Findings
Hypocalcemia
Hyperphosphatemia
Decreased serum parathyroid hormone concentration

Electrocardiographic Findings
Deep, wide T waves
Prolonged QT interval
Bradycardia

Pheochromocytoma

CLINICAL FINDINGS
Intermittent weakness
Intermittent collapse
Panting
Tachypnea
Tachycardia
Lethargy
Inappetence
Cardiac arrhythmias

Weak pulses
Vomiting
Diarrhea
Weight loss
Muscle wasting
Polyuria/polydipsia
Abdominal distension
Rear limb edema
Pale mucous membranes
Abdominal pain
Hemorrhage (epistaxis, surgical incision sites)
Palpable abdominal mass

Pituitary Dwarfism

CLINICAL FINDINGS

Musculoskeletal Signs

Stunted growth
Delayed growth plate closure
Thin skeleton
Immature facial features
Square, chunky contour as adult
Bone deformities
Delayed dental eruption

Dermatologic Signs

Soft, wooly haircoat
Lack of guard hairs
Alopecia; bilaterally symmetric trunk, neck, and
    proximal extremities
Hyperpigmentation
Thin, fragile skin
Wrinkles
Scales
Comedones
Papules
Pyoderma
Seborrhea sicca
Retention of secondary hairs

Reproductive Signs

Testicular atrophy
Flaccid penile sheath
Failure to have estrous cycles

Other Signs
Mental dullness
Shrill, puppy-like bark
Signs of secondary hypothyroidism
Signs of secondary adrenal insufficiency

Thyroid Disease

HYPERTHYROIDISM, FELINE—CLINICAL FINDINGS
Clinical Signs
Weight loss/thin body condition
Polyphagia
Hyperactivity
Palpable thyroid nodule (goiter)
Tachycardia
Vomiting
Cardiac murmur
Premature beats
Gallop rhythm
Aggressiveness
Panting
Pacing
Restlessness
Increased nail growth
Alopecia
Polyuria/polydipsia
Diarrhea
Increased fecal volume
Muscle weakness
Congestive heart failure (CHF)
Dyspnea
Ventroflexion of neck
Unkempt coat/alopecia
Tremor
Weakness

HYPOTHYROIDISM, CANINE—CLINICAL FINDINGS
Clinical Signs
Lethargy/exercise intolerance
Weight gain
Cold intolerance
Mental dullness
Dermatologic signs

- Alopecia
- Superficial pyoderma
- Seborrhea sicca or oleosa
- Dry, scaly skin
- Changes in haircoat quality and color
- Hyperkeratosis
- Hyperpigmentation
- Comedones
- Hypertrichosis
- Ceruminous otitis
- Myxedema (cutaneous mucinosis)
- Poor wound healing
- Slow regrowth of hair

Reproductive abnormalities
- Male: decreased libido, testicular atrophy, hypospermia
- Female: delayed estrus, silent estrus, failure to cycle, abortion, small litters, uterine inertia

Peripheral neuropathies
- Generalized peripheral neuropathies
- Specific peripheral neuropathies (especially cranial nerves, facial, trigeminal, vestibulcochlear)

Cerebral dysfunction (myxedema coma [rare])

Cardiovascular signs
- Sinus bradycardia, weak apex beat, low QRS voltages, inverted T waves, hypercholesterolemia leading to atherosclerosis (rare)

Ocular abnormalities (corneal lipidosis, corneal ulceration, uveitis, secondary glaucoma, lipemia retinalis, retinal detachment, and keratoconjunctivitis sicca reported, but causal relationship not proven)

Clinicopathologic Changes
Nonregenerative anemia
Hypercholesterolemia
Hypertriglyceridemia
Mild increases in hepatic enzymes

Section IV

Gastroenterologic Disorders

Dental and Oral Cavity Diseases

DIFFERENTIAL DIAGNOSIS

Trauma

Fractures

- Crown
- Root
- Mandibule
- Maxillar

Avulsion

Pulp injury

Temporomandibular luxation?

Caries

Feline Odontoclastic Resorptive Lesions (FORLs)

Periodontal Disease

Gingivitis

Gingival recession

Bone loss, osteomyelitis

Tooth loss

Tooth Root Abscess

Oronasal Fistula

Stomatitis (Faucitis, Glossitis, Pharyngitis)

Feline immunodeficiency virus, feline leukemia virus
Feline calicivirus, feline herpesvirus
Uremia
Trauma (foreign objects, caustic agents, electric cord bite)
Autoimmune disease (pemphigus, lupus)
Feline lymphocytic/plasmacytic gingivitis/pharyngitis

Neoplasia

Malignant

Fibrosarcoma
Squamous cell carcinoma
Melanoma

Benign

Epulis
- Fibromatous
- Acanthomatous

Eosinophilic Granuloma Complex

Sialocele

Salivary Gland Disease

DIFFERENTIAL DIAGNOSIS

Salivary Neoplasia (more common in cats than dogs)

Adenocarcinoma
Squamous cell carcinoma
Undifferentiated sarcoma
Mucoepidermoid tumor
Malignant mixed tumor
Sarcoma
Acinic cell carcinoma
Adenoid cystic carcinoma

Salivary Mucocele

Sublingual gland most commonly

Sialoadenitis

Sialoadenosis

Esophageal Disease

DIFFERENTIAL DIAGNOSIS
Congenital
Obstruction
Persistent right aortic arch
Persistent right or left subclavian artery
Other vascular ring anomaly

Idiopathic

Acquired
Obstruction
Foreign body
Cicatrix/stricture
Neoplasia
- Carcinoma
- *Spirocerca lupi*–induced sarcoma
- Leiomyoma of lower esophageal sphincter
- Extraesophageal neoplasia
  - Thyroid carcinoma
  - Pulmonary carcinoma
Achalasia of lower esophageal sphincter (rare)
Gastroesophageal intussusception (rare)

Weakness
Myasthenia (generalized or localized)
Hypoadrenocorticism
Esophagitis
Persistent vomiting
Hiatal hernia
Gastroesophageal reflux
Caustic ingestion

Spirocerca lupi infection

Myopathies/neuropathies
Hypothyroidism
Systemic lupus erythematosus (SLE)
Others

Miscellaneous Causes
Lead poisoning
Chagas' disease
Canine distemper

Dermatomyositis (principally in Collies)
Dysautonomia

Idiopathic

Stomach Disorders

DIFFERENTIAL DIAGNOSIS
Gastritis
Acute Gastritis
Dietary indiscretion
Dietary intolerance or allergy
Foreign body
Drugs and toxins (nonsteroidal antiinflammatory
drugs [NSAIDs], corticosteroids, antibiotics, plants,
cleaners, bleach, heavy metals)
Systemic disease (uremia, hepatic disease,
hypoadrenocorticism)
Parasites (*Ollulanus* spp., *Physaloptera* spp.)
Bacterial (bacterial toxins, *Helicobacter* spp.)

Hemorrhagic Gastroenteritis

Chronic Gastritis
Lymphocytic/plasmacytic gastritis
Eosinophilic gastritis
Granulomatous gastritis
Atrophic gastritis

Gastric Outflow Obstruction/Gastric Stasis
Benign muscular pyloric hypertrophy (pyloric stenosis)
Gastric antral mucosal hypertrophy
Foreign body
Idiopathic gastric hypomotility
Bilious vomiting syndrome

Gastric Ulceration/Erosion
Iatrogenic
NSAIDs
Corticosteroids
NSAID/corticosteroid combinations

Foreign Body

Stress Ulceration
Hypovolemic shock

Septic shock
After gastric dilatation/volvulus
- Neurogenic shock
Hyperacidity
- Mast cell tumor
- Gastrinoma (rare)
Other causes
- Hepatic disease
- Renal disease
- Hypoadrenocorticism
- Inflammatory disease

Infiltrative Disease
Neoplasia
Inflammatory bowel disease
Pythiosis (young dogs, southeastern United States)

Gastric Dilatation/Volvulus

CAUSES OF ACUTE ABDOMEN
Gastrointestinal (GI) Causes
Pancreatitis
Gastroenteritis (parvoviral, bacterial, toxic, hemorrhagic
gastroenteritis, etc.)
Gastric dilatation/volvulus
Intestinal obstruction/intussusception
Colitis
Obstipation
Necrosis, rupture, ulceration, or perforation of GI tract
Surgical wound dehiscence
Mesenteric torsion
Duodenocolic ligament entrapment

Hepatobiliary Causes
Acute hepatitis/cholangiohepatitis
Biliary obstruction
Necrotizing cholecystitis
Hepatic abscess
Bile peritonitis
Liver lobe torsion

Urogenital Causes
Urethral obstruction/rupture
Pyelonephritis
Cystic calculi
Prostatitis/prostatic abscess
Dystocia

    Pyometra/uterine rupture
    Renal abscess
    Testicular torsion
    Uroabdomen
    Vaginal rupture

Other Causes
    Penetrating wound, crush injury
    Hemoabdomen (parenchymatous organ rupture)
    Neoplasia
    Splenic torsion/abscess
    Strangulated hernia
    Pansteatitis
    Retroperitoneal hemorrhage
    Evisceration
    Surgical contamination

Small Intestinal Disease

CLINICAL FINDINGS
    Diarrhea
    Vomiting
    Inappetence/anorexia
    Weight loss
    Dehydration
    Hematemesis
    Melena
    Polyphagia
    Coprophagia
    Abdominal distension
    Abdominal pain
    Borborygmus/flatulence
    Ascites
    Edema
    Shock
    Halitosis
    Polydipsia
    Ileus

DIFFERENTIAL DIAGNOSIS
    Acute Diarrhea
        Acute enteritis
        Dietary indiscretion

Infectious Diarrhea

Canine parvoviral enteritis
Clostridial disease
Feline parvoviral enteritis (panleukopenia)
Canine coronaviral enteritis
Feline coronaviral enteritis
Feline leukemia virus–associated panleukopenia
Feline immunodeficiency virus–associated diarrhea
Salmon poisoning (*Neorickettsia helminthoeca*)
Campylobacteriosis
Salmonellosis
Histoplasmosis
Miscellaneous bacteria *(Yersinia enterocolitica, Aeromonas hydrophila, Plesiomonas shigelloides)*
Prototothecosis (algae)

Alimentary Tract Parasites

Roundworms (*Toxocara* spp.)
Hookworms (*Ancylostoma, Uncinaria* spp.)
Tapeworms (*Dipylidium caninum, Taenia* spp., *Mesocestoides* spp.)
Strongyloides stercoralis (in puppies)
Coccidiosis
Cryptosporidia
Giardiasis

Maldigestive Disease

Exocrine pancreatic insufficiency

Malabsorptive Disease

Lymphocytic/plasmacytic enteritis
Canine eosinophilic gastroenteritis
Feline eosinophilic enteritis/hypereosinophilic syndrome
Granulomatous enteritis
Immunoproliferative enteropathy in Basenjis
Enteropathy in Shar-Peis
Antibiotic-responsive enteropathy

Protein-losing enteropathy

Intestinal lymphangectasia
Protein-losing enteropathy in Soft-Coated Wheaton Terriers

Intestinal Obstruction

Simple intestinal obstruction
Incarcerated intestinal obstruction

Mesenteric torsion/volvulus
Linear foreign object

Intussusception
Ileocolic
Jejunojejunal

Short-Bowel Syndrome

Neoplasia
Alimentary lymphoma
Intestinal adenocarcinoma
Intestinal leiomyoma/leiomyosarcoma

BREED SUSCEPTIBILITIES, DOGS
Basenji: lymphocytic/plasmacytic enteritis
(immunoproliferative disease)
Beagle: cobalamin deficiency
Border Collie: cobalamin deficiency
German Shepherd: idiopathic antibiotic-responsive small
intestinal disease, inflammatory bowel disease
(lymphoplasmacytic, eosinophilic)
Giant Schnauzer: defective cobalamin absorption
Irish Setter: gluten-sensitive enteropathy
Lundehund: lymphangiectasia
Retrievers: dietary allergy
Rottweiler: increased susceptibility to parvoviral enteritis
Soft-Coated Wheaton Terrier: protein-losing
enteropathy/nephropathy
Shar-Pei: lymphocytic/plasmacytic enteritis, cobalamin
deficiency
Yorkshire Terrier: lymphangiectasia
Toy breeds: hemorrhagic gastroenteritis

Large Intestinal Disease

DIFFERENTIAL DIAGNOSIS
Inflammation of Large Intestine
Acute colitis/proctitis
Chronic colitis
• Lymphocytic/plasmacytic colitis
• Eosinophilic enterocolitis
• Chronic ulcerative colitis
• Histiocytic ulcerative colitis (Boxers)
Irritable bowel syndrome

Dietary Intolerance or Food Allergy

Parasites
  Whipworms (*Trichuris* spp.)
  Tritrichomonas spp. (cats)
  Giardiasis
  Hookworms (*Ancylostoma* spp.)
  Heterobilharzia americanum

Bacterial Colitis
  Clostridial colitis
  Campylobacter colitis
  Escherichia coli
  Salmonella spp.
  Brachispira pilosicoli

Fungal colitis
  Histoplasmosis
  Pythiosis

Viral Colitis
  Feline leukemia virus (FeLV)
  Infections secondary to FeLV and feline
    immunodeficiency virus (FIV)

Algae (*Prototheca* spp.)

Cecocolic Intussusception

Rectal Prolapse

Neoplasms of Large Intestine
  Adenocarcinoma
  Lymphoma
  Rectal polyps

Pythiosis

Constipation
  Pelvic canal obstruction caused by malaligned healing of
    pelvic fractures
  Benign rectal stricture
  Dietary indiscretion leading to constipation
  Idiopathic megacolon

Ileus

CAUSES

Physical
Intestinal obstruction
Overdistension by aerophagia

Metabolic
Uremia
Hypokalemia
Endotoxemia

Functional
Abdominal surgery
Inflammatory disease
Peritonitis
Parvovirus
Pancreatitis
Ischemia

Neuromuscular
Anticholinergic drugs
Spinal cord injury
Visceral myopathies
Dysautonomia

Malabsorptive Diseases

CAUSES
Food intolerance or allergy
Parasiticism
• Giardiasis
Bacterial overgrowth
Inflammatory bowel disease
• Lymphocytic/plasmacytic enteritis
• Eosinophilic enteritis
• Idiopathic villous atrophy
• Purulent enteritis
Gastrointestinal lymphoma
Lymphangiectasia
Obstruction caused by neoplasia, infection, or inflammation
Portal hypertension
Pythiosis
Exocrine pancreatic insufficiency

Cholestatic liver disease/biliary obstruction
Brush border enzyme deficiencies
Brush border transport protein deficiencies
Hyperthyroidism
Gastric hypersecretion

Perianal Disease

DIFFERENTIAL DIAGNOSIS
Perineal hernia
Perianal fistulas
Anal sacculitis
Abscessed anal sac
Anal sac (apocrine gland) adenocarcinoma
Perianal gland tumors
- Adenoma (common)
- Adenosarcoma (rare)

Protein-Losing Enteropathy

DIFFERENTIAL DIAGNOSIS
Gastrointestinal Hemorrhage
Hemorrhagic gastroenteritis
Ulceration
Neoplasia

Endoparasites
Giardia spp.
Ancylostoma spp.
Coccidia
Others

Inflammation
Lymphocytic/plasmacytic
Eosinophilic
Granulomatous

Infection
Parvovirus
Salmonellosis
Histoplasmosis
Phycomycosis

Structural
  Intussusception

Neoplasia
  Lymphosarcoma

Lymphangiectasia
  Primary lymphatic disorder
  Venous hypertension
  Hepatic cirrhosis

Fecal Incontinence

CAUSES
  Nonneurologic Disease
    Colorectal Disease
      Inflammatory bowel disease
      Neoplasia
      Constipation

    Anorectal Disease
      Perianal fistula
      Neoplasia
      Surgery (anal sacculectomy, perianal herniorrhaphy,
        rectal resection and anastomosis)

    Miscellaneous
      Decreased mentation
      Old age
      Severe diarrhea
      Irritable bowel disease

  Neurologic Disease
    Sacral Spinal Cord Disease
      Diskospondylitis
      Neoplasia
      Degenerative myelopathy
      Congenital vertebral malformation
      Sacrococcygeal hypoplasia of Manx cats
      Sacral fracture
      Sacrococcygeal subluxation
      Lumbosacral instability
      Meningomyelocele
      Viral meningomyelitis

Peripheral Neuropathy
  Trauma
  Penetrating wounds
  Repair of perineal hernia
  Perineal urethrostomy
  Hypothyroidism
  Diabetes mellitus
  Dysautonomia

Hematologic Disorders

Anemia

HEMOLYTIC ANEMIA

Causes/Triggers of Immune-Mediated Hemolytic Anemia

Infection

Viral

Feline leukemia virus (FeLV), feline immunodeficiency virus (FIV), feline peritonitis virus (FIP), chronic upper respiratory or gastrointestinal (GI) disease

Bacterial

Leptospirosis, *Mycoplasma haemophilus* infection, acute and chronic infections (e.g., abscess, pyometra, diskospondylitis)

Parasitic

Babesiosis, leishmaniasis, dirofilariasis, ehrlichiosis, *Ancylostoma caninum* infection, bartonellosis

Immune Disorders

Systemic lupus erythematosus (SLE)
Hypothyroidism
Primary and secondary immunodeficiencies

Drugs

Vaccines
Sulfonamides
Methimazole

Procainamide
Cephalosporins
Penicillins
Propylthiouracil

Oxidants
Acetaminophen
Phenothiazines
Vitamin K
Methylene blue
Methionine
Propylene glycol

Neoplasia
Leukemias
Lymphoma
Multiple myeloma
Solid tumors

Genetic Predisposition
American Cocker Spaniel (most common breed),
English Springer Spaniel, Old English Sheepdog,
Irish Setter, Poodle, Dachshund

Differentiating Blood Loss from Hemolytic Anemia
Blood Loss
Serum or plasma protein concentration normal to low
Clinical evidence of hemorrhage
No icterus, hemoglobinemia, spherocytosis,
hemosiderinuria, autoagglutination, splenomegaly,
or red blood cell (RBC) changes
Negative direct Coombs' test

Hemolysis
Serum or plasma protein concentration normal
to high
Rarely clinical evidence of hemorrhage
Icterus common
Hemoglobinuria
Spherocytosis
Hemosiderinuria
Autoagglutination sometimes seen
Direct Coombs' test usually positive
Splenomegaly
RBC changes numerous

NONREGENERATIVE ANEMIA
Differential Diagnosis
Anemia of Chronic Disease
Erythropoietin-Related Conditions
Renal disease
Hypothyroidism
Hypoadrenocorticism
Panhypopituitarism
Growth hormone deficiency
Reduced oxygen requirement
Increased oxygen release

Iron Deficiency Anemia
Chronic inflammation
Chronic hemorrhage
Dietary iron deficiency

Marrow Disorders
Toxic Red Cell Aplasia
Estrogen related
Phenylbutazone related
Other drugs

Hyperestrogenism (Iatrogenic, Neoplastic)

Infection
Feline leukemia virus (FeLV)
Feline immunodeficiency virus (FIV)
Parvovirus
Ehrlichiosis
Babesiosis
Mycoplasma haemofelis
Endotoxemia

Immunotherapy

Myelofibrosis
Feline leukemia virus (FeLV) infection
Pyruvate kinase deficiency anemia
Idiopathic

Myelophthistic Disease
Acute leukemias
Chronic leukemias
Multiple myeloma
Lymphoma
Systemic mast cell disease

Malignant Histiocytosis
Metastatic carcinoma
Histoplasmosis

Myelodysplasia
Idiopathic
FeLV/FIV
Preleukemic syndrome

Pure Red Cell Aplasia

Ineffective Erythropoiesis
Macrocytic (rare)
Intrinsic marrow disease
Vitamin B_{12} deficiency
Folic acid deficiency

Normocytic
Myelofibrosis
Intrinsic erythroid disease

Microcytic
Iron deficiency
Globin or porphyrin deficiency

Time Related
Hemolysis or hemorrhage (during the first
3-5 days)

Diagnosis
Nonregenerative Anemias without Other Cytopenias
Examine bone marrow.

Severe Erythroid Hypoplasia
Pure red cell aplasia

Normal to Mild Erythroid Hypoplasia
Inflammatory disease
Renal disease
Neoplasia
Hepatic disease
Hypothyroidism
Hypoadrenocorticism

Hypercellular Bone Marrow
Less than 30% blast forms: consider
myelodysplastic syndrome.
Greater than 30% blast forms: consider
hemopoietic neoplasia.

Nonregenerative Anemias with Leukopenia and/or Thrombocytopenia

Examine bone marrow.

Panhypoplasia
Aplastic anemia

Disease Determined by Core Biopsy
Myelonecrosis
Myelofibrosis

Hypercellular Bone Marrow
Less than 30% blast forms: myelodysplastic syndrome
More than 30% blast forms: hemopoietic neoplasia

REGENERATIVE ANEMIA

Differential Diagnosis

Hemolysis
Immune mediated
- Intravascular
- Extravascular

Blood Loss Anemia
Trauma
Coagulopathy
- Clotting factor deficiency
- Disseminated intravascular coagulation (DIC)
- Platelet disorders
- Anticoagulant rodenticides
Endoparasites
GI blood loss
Severe ectoparasites (fleas)

Oxidative Injury (Heinz Body)
Onion ingestion
Acetaminophen (cats)
Zinc ingestion (pennies minted after 1982, zinc oxide ointment, zinc-plated bolts and screws)
Benzocaine ingestion (dogs)
D-L Methionine (cats)
Phenolic compounds (mothballs)
Phenazopyridine (cats)

Erythrocytic Parasites
Haemobartonella spp.
Babesia spp.
Cytauxzoon spp.

Fragmentation (Microangiopathic)
Disseminated intravascular coagulation (DIC)
Heartworm disease
Hemangiosarcoma
Vasculitis
Hemolytic-uremic syndrome
Diabetes mellitus

Other
Copper toxicity
Neonatal isoerythrolysis
Hereditary nonspherocytic hemolytic anemia
Pyruvate kinase deficiency
Feline porphyria
Hemolysis in Abyssinian and Somali cats

Coagulopathies, Inherited and Acquired

DIFFERENTIAL DIAGNOSIS
Inherited Clotting Factor Deficiencies
Hemophilia A (factor VIII deficiency)
Hemophilia B (factor IX deficiency)
Factor XII deficiency (Hageman trait)
Vitamin K–dependent factor deficiency: factors II, VII, IX, X (Devon Rex cats)
Factor I: hypofibrinogenemia or dysfibrinogenemia (St. Bernard, Borzoi)
Factor II: hypoprothrombinemia (Boxer, Otterhound, English Cocker Spaniel)
Factor VII: hypoproconvertinemia (Beagle, Malamute, Boxer, Bulldog, Miniature Schnauzer)
Factor X deficiency (Cocker Spaniel, Parson Russell Terrier)
Hemophilia C (factor XI deficiency: English Springer Spaniel, Great Pyrenees, Kerry Blue Terrier)
Prekallikrein deficiency (Fletcher factor)

Acquired Clotting Factor Deficiency
Liver disease
• Decreased clotting factor production
• Qualitative disorders
Cholestasis
Vitamin K antagonists
Autoimmune disease (lupus anticoagulant)
Disseminated intravascular coagulation (DIC)

Leukocyte Disorders

DIFFERENTIAL DIAGNOSIS

Pelger-Huët anomaly (many breeds of dogs and cats)
- Neutrophil function not altered

Chédiak-Higashi syndrome (blue smoke-colored Persian cats)

Canine leukocyte adhesion deficiency: fatal defect (Irish Setter and Irish Setter crosses)

Cyclic hemopoiesis (cyclic neutropenia): fatal defect (gray Collies)

Birman cat neutrophil granulation anomaly: neutophil function not altered

Hypereosinophilic syndrome (cats): may eventually be fatal

Severe combined immunodeficiency of Parson Russell Terriers: fatal defect

Canine X-linked severe combined immunodeficiency: fatal defect (many breeds)

Defective neutrophil function in Doberman Pinscher: need frequent antimicrobial therapy

Immunodeficiency of Shar-Peis

Immunodeficiency of Weimaraners

Lysosomal storage diseases (many types described, all rare, many breeds)

Platelet Dysfunction

DIFFERENTIAL DIAGNOSIS

Acquired Platelet Dysfunction

Drugs

Prostaglandin inhibitors (NSAIDs)
Vaccines
Antibiotics
Antifungals
Phenothiazines
Aminophylline
Diltiazem
Isoproterenol

Secondary to Disease

Renal disease
Liver disease
Myeloproliferative disorders

Systemic lupus erythematosus (SLE)
Dysproteinemias

Hereditary
Von Willebrand's disease (many breeds)
Canine thrombopathia (Basset Hound, Foxhound, Spitz)
Canine thrombasthenic thrombopathia (Otterhound,
Great Pyrenees)
Collagen deficiency diseases/Ehler-Danlos syndrome
(many breeds)

Splenitis/Splenomegaly

DIFFERENTIAL DIAGNOSIS FOR SPLENOMEGALY
Splenic Mass (Asymmetric Splenomegaly)
Nodular hyperplasia
Hematoma
Neoplasia
- Hemangiosarcoma
- Hemangioma
- Leiomyosarcoma
- Fibrosarcoma
- Leiomyoma
- Myelolipoma
Abscess
Extramedullary hematopoiesis
Granuloma

Uniform splenomegaly
Congestion
Drugs
Portal hypertension
Right-sided heart failure
Splenic torsion

Hyperplasia
Chronic infection
Inflammatory bowel disease
Systemic lupus erythematosus (SLE)
Polycythemia vera

Extramedullary Hematopoiesis
Chronic anemia
Immune-mediated hemolytic anemia
Immune-mediated thrombocytopenia
Neoplasia

Neoplasia
Lymphoma
Systemic mastocytosis
Metastatic neoplasia
Multiple myeloma
Metastatic neoplasia
Acute and chronic leukemias
Malignant histiocytosis

Nonneoplastic Infiltrative Disease
Amyloidosis

Inflammation
Suppurative
Sepsis
Bacterial endocarditis
Infectious canine hepatitis
Foreign body
Penetrating wounds

Granulomatous
Cryptococcosis
Histoplasmosis
Mycobacteriosis
Leishmaniasis

Pyogranulomatous
Feline infectious peritonitis (FIP)
Blastomycosis
Sporotrichosis

Eosinophilic
Eosinophilic gastroenteritis
Hypereosinophilic syndrome
Neoplasia

Lymphoplasmacytic
Ehrlichiosis
Hemotropic mycoplasmosis
Lymphoplasmacytic enteritis
Pyometra
Brucellosis

Necrotic Tissue
Torsion
Necrotic center of neoplasms
Infectious canine hepatitis
Tularemia
Salmonellosis

INFECTIOUS CAUSES
> **Viral**
>> Feline leukemia virus (FeLV)
>> Feline immunodeficiency virus (FIV)
>> Feline infectious peritonitis (FIP)
>> Infectious canine hepatitis
>
> **Bacterial**
>> Canine brucellosis
>> Mycoplasmosis
>> Borreliosis
>> Plague
>> Tularemia
>> Streptococcosis
>> Staphylococcosis
>> Salmonellosis
>> *Francisella* infection
>> Endotoxemia
>
> **Fungal**
>> Cryptococcosis
>> Histoplasmosis
>> Blastomycosis
>
> **Rickettsial**
>> Ehrlichiosis
>> Rocky Mountain spotted fever
>> Q fever (*Coxiella burnetii*)
>> *Mycoplasma haemofelis*
>
> **Protozoal**
>> Toxoplasmosis
>> Cytauxzoonosis (cat)
>> Babesiosis (*Babesia canis* and *B. gibsoni*)
>> Leishmaniasis (dog)

Thrombocytopenia

DIFFERENTIAL DIAGNOSIS
> **Increased Platelet**
>> **Destruction/Sequestration/Utilization**
>> Immune-mediated thrombocytopenia
>> Drug-induced thrombocytopenia
>> Microangiopathy
>> Disseminated intravascular coagulation

Neoplasia
Live viral vaccine–induced thrombocytopenia
Hemolytic uremic syndrome/thrombotic
    thrombocytopenic purpura
Vasculitis
Splenomegaly
Splenic torsion
Endotoxemia
Acute hepatic necrosis
Hemorrhage

Decreased Platelet Production

Drug-induced megakaryocytic hypoplasia (estrogen,
    phenylbutazone, melphalan, lomustine, β-lactams)
Myelophthisis
Idiopathic bone marrow aplasia
Retroviral infection (FeLV/FIV)
Immune-mediated megakaryocytic hypoplasia
Cyclic thrombocytopenia
Ehrlichiosis

Immunologic and Immune-Mediated Disorders

Autoimmune Skin Diseases
Immune-Mediated Disease
Immune System Components
Systemic Lupus Erythematosus (SLE)

Autoimmune Skin Diseases

DIFFERENTIAL DIAGNOSIS

Generalized Pustular/Crusting Dermatosis

Pemphigus foliaceus (PF) (nose, ear pinna, and footpad typically affected)

Pemphigus-like drug reactions (nasal and footpad lesions may be absent)

Others: rare presentation—systemic lupus erythematosus (SLE), sterile eosinophilic pustulosis, linear immunoglobulin A (IgA) pustular dermatosis, subcorneal pustular dermatosis

Focal Pustular/Crusting Dermatosis

Face, footpads: PF

Face and ears only: PF (early), pemphigus erythematosus (PE), drug eruptions, lupus erythematosus

Nasal only: discoid lupus erythematosus (DLE), PF (early), PE

Mucocutaneous and Mucosal Ulcerations

Pemphigus vulgaris (may also have oral lesions)

Mucous membrane bullous pemphigoid

Epidermolysis bullosa acquisita

Erythema multiforme (target lesions, cutaneous lesions)

Bullous SLE

Drug reactions

Linear IgA bullous dermatosis, toxic epidermal necrolysis (rare)

Nonmucosal Ulcerations (Axillae, Inguinae, Pinnae, Other Haired Areas)
Bullous pemphigoid
Epidermolysis bullosa acquisita
Linear IgA bullous dermatosis
Bullous SLE
Canine vesicular cutaneous lupus erythematosus
(idiopathic ulcerative dermatosis of Collies, Shetland
Sheepdogs)
Erythema multiforme (EM)
Toxic epidermal necrolysis
Drug eruptions
Pemphigus vulgaris

Depigmenting Skin Diseases
Nasal only: DLE, vitiligo-like syndrome,
uveodermatologic syndrome, early PF or PE
Nose, footpad, lip, eyelid, mucocutaneous area:
uveodermatologic syndrome (uveitis also)
Haircoat or skin: idiopathic leukotrichia or leukoderma

Miscellaneous
Focal alopecia: alopecia areata, rabies vaccine, focal
vasculitis
Widespread noninflammatory alopecia: alopecia areata,
pseudopelade
Erythematous target lesions: erythema multiforme
Nodular ulcerative lesions: nodular panniculitis
Purpura, hemorrhage, punched-out lesions, ear margin
necrosis, dependent edema: vasculitis

Immune-Mediated Disease

LABORATORY DIAGNOSIS
Direct Coombs' Test
Immune-mediated hemolytic anemia
Hemolytic anemia in systemic lupus erythematosus (SLE)

Antiplatelet Antibodies
Immune-mediated thrombocytopenia

Antinuclear Antibody
SLE
Chronic antigenic stimulation

Rheumatoid Factor
Rheumatoid arthritis (RA)

Direct Immunofluorescence
Antibody-complement deposition

DIFFERENTIAL DIAGNOSIS FOR IMMUNE-MEDIATED ARTHRITIS

Erosive Immune-Mediated Arthritides
RA (dog, rarely in cat)
Periosteal proliferative polyarthritis (cat, rarely in dog)

Nonerosive Immune-Mediated Arthritides
Idiopathic polyarthritis
- Type I: uncomplicated idiopathic arthritis (most common)
- Type II: idiopathic arthritis associated with infection remote from joints—respiratory tract, tonsils, conjunctiva (chlamydia in cats), urinary tract, uterus, skin, oral cavity
- Type III: idiopathic arthritis associated with gastroenteritis
- Type IV: idiopathic arthritis associated with malignant neoplasia—squamous cell carcinoma, heart base tumor, leiomyoma, mammary carcinoma, myeloproliferative disease (cats)

SLE
Drug-induced polyarthritis
- Sulfas, lincomycin, erythromycin, cephalosporins, penicillins, trimethoprim-sulfa (especially Doberman Pinscher)

Vaccination reaction
Polyarthritis/polymyositis syndrome
Polyarthritis/meningitis syndrome
Familial renal amyloidosis in Chinese Shar-Peis
Polyarthritis in adolescent Akitas
Polyarthritis nodosa (inflammatory condition of small arteries—histopathologic diagnosis)

Immune System Components

FUNCTION
Humoral Immunity
B Lymphocytes and Plasma Cells
Production of immunoglobulins

Cellular Immunity
T Lymphocytes
Production of lymphokines
Helper T cells
- Stimulate immune reactivity
Suppressor T cells
- Suppress immune reactivity
Antibody-dependent cell-mediated cytotoxity
Natural killer cells
- Direct cytotoxicity

Phagocytic Cells
Mononuclear Phagocytic Cells
Antigen presentation
Phagocytosis of particles

Neutrophils and Eosinophils
Phagocytosis of particles
Antibody-dependent cell-mediated cytotoxicity

Systemic Lupus Erythematosus (SLE)

ORGANS AND TISSUES AFFECTED
Red blood cells
- Immune-mediated hemolytic anemia
- Pure red cell aplasia
Platelets
- Immune-mediated thrombocytopenia
Glomeruli
- Glomerulonephritis
Synovium
- Nonerosive polyarthritis
Blood vessels
- Vasculitis
Epidermis
- Dermatitis

Neutrophils
- Immune-mediated neutrophilia

Clotting factors
- Coagulopathy

Central nervous system
- Seizures, focal signs

Skeletal muscle/nerve end plate
- Polymyositis
- Polyneuritis
- Myasthenia gravis

CRITERIA FOR DIAGNOSIS IN DOGS AND CATS

SLE is diagnosed when three or more of the following criteria are manifested simultaneously or at any time:

Antinuclear antibodies (ANAs)
- Abnormal ANA titer in the absence of drugs or infectious or neoplastic conditions known to be associated with abnormal titers

Cutaneous lesions
- Depigmentation, erythema, erosions, ulcerations, crusts, scaling, with biopsy findings consistent with SLE

Oral ulcers
- Oral or nasopharyngeal ulceration, usually painless

Arthritis
- Nonerosive, nonseptic arthritis involving two or more peripheral joints

Renal disorders
- Glomerulonephritis or persistent proteinuria in the absence of urinary tract infection

Anemia/thrombocytopenia
- Hemolytic anemia/thrombocytopenia in the absence of offending drugs

Leukopenia
- Low total white cell count

Polymyositis or myocarditis
- Inflammatory disease of skeletal or cardiac muscles

Serositis
- Presence of a nonseptic inflammatory cavity effusion (abdominal, pleural, or pericardial)

Neurologic disorders
- Seizures or psychosis in the absence of known disorders

Antiphospholipids
- Prolongation of activated partial thromboplastin time (APTT) that fails to correct with a 1:1 mixture of patient's and normal plasma, in the absence of heparin or fibrin degradation products (FDP)

Infectious Disease

Bacterial Infections, Systemic

DIFFERENTIAL DIAGNOSIS

Leptospirosis

Hepatic dysfunction, renal dysfunction, fever, anterior uveitis, icterus

Coagulation abnormalities, vomiting/diarrhea, icterus, polyuria/polydipsia

Borreliosis (Lyme Disease)

Fever, inappetence/lethargy, lymphadenopathy, polyarthritis

Glomerulonephritis/acute, progressive renal failure, mild dermatologic lesions

Meningitis/encephalitis (rare), myocarditis

Mycobacteriosis

Often asymptomatic, skin lesions, dermal nodules, draining tracts, lymphadenopathy, bronchopneumonia, pulmonary nodules, hilar lymphadenopathy, vomiting, diarrhea secondary to intestinal malabsorption, feline leprosy

Brucellosis (Dogs)

Fever, lymphadenopathy, epididymitis, scrotal enlargement, scrotal dermatitis, infertility

Abortion in pregnant bitches, diskospondylitis

Rarely uveitis, glomerulonephritis, meningoencephalitis

Tetanus
Localized tetanus, especially cats; stiffness in a muscle of limb
Stiff gait, outstretched or dorsally curved tails, extreme muscle rigidity
Ears erect, lips drawn back (sardonic grin), protrusion of globe, enophthalmos
Trismus (lockjaw), laryngeal spasm, regurgitation, megaesophagus leading to aspiration pneumonia

Botulism
Generalized lower motor neuron and parasympathetic dysfunction
Quadriplegia, megaesophagus, respiratory paralysis; may lead to death

Feline Plague *(Yersinia pestis)*
Spread by fleas
May show signs of bubonic, septicemic, and pneumonic plague

Mycoplasmosis/Ureaplasmosis (Cats)
Conjunctivitis, sneezing, mucopurulent nasal discharge, coughing, dyspnea, fever, lameness, swollen joints, subcutaneous abscessation

NOMENCLATURE OF OBLIGATE INTRACELLULAR BACTERIAL PATHOGENS
Rickettsioses (Spotted Fever Group Rickettsiae)
Rickettsia rickettsii (the type species), *R. africae, R. akari, R. australis, R. conorii, R. montana, R. parkeri, R. rhipicephali, R. sibirica,* and *R. felis*
Species of the following tick genera transmit spotted-fever group agents: *Dermacentor, Rhipicephalus, Haemaphysalis,* and *Amblyomma*

Ehrlichiosis (Canine)
Ehrlichia canis, E. chaffeensis, E. ewingii, E. muris, and *E. ruminantium*

Anaplasmosis (Canine and Feline)
Anaplasma phagocytophilium
Anaplasma platys (canine cyclic thrombocytopenia: mildly pathogenic)

Bartonellosis, Canine

CLINICAL FINDINGS
Many species of *Bartonella* are suspected to cause disease in dogs (e.g., *B. vinsonii, B. henselae, B. clarridgeae, B. elizabethae*)
Fever
Endocarditis
Intermittent lameness
Bone pain
Granulomatous lymphadenitis
Dermatologic lesions/cutaneous vasculitis
Anterior uveitis
Polyarthritis
Meningoencephalitis
Immune-mediated hemolytic anemia
Thrombocytopenia
Eosinophilia
Peliosis hepatitis
Granulomatous hepatitis
Chronic weight loss

Ehrlichiosis, Canine

CLINICAL FINDINGS
  Acute
    Fever
    Anorexia/weight loss
    Serous or purulent oculonasal discharge
    Lymphadenopathy
    Dyspnea
    History of recent or present tick bite
    Thrombocytopenia
    Leukopenia followed by leukocytosis and monocytosis
    Low-grade nonregenerative anemia, unless hemorrhage
    Variable *Ehrlichia* titer, polymerase chain reaction (PCR)
      positive

  Subclinical
    No clinical abnormalities apparent
    Hyperglobulinemia, thrombocytopenia, neutropenia,
      lymphocytosis, monocytosis
    Positive *Ehrlichia* titer, PCR positive

Chronic

Depression

Pale mucous membranes

Weight loss

Abdominal pain

Splenomegaly

Epistaxis, retinal hemorrhage, other examples of hemorrhage

Lymphadenopathy

Stiffness, swollen/painful joints

Hepatomegaly

Dyspnea, interstitial or alveolar lung infiltrates

Perivascular retinitis, hyphema, retinal detachment, anterior uveitis, corneal edema

Seizures, paresis, meningeal pain, cranial nerve deficits

Arrhythmias

Polyuria/polydipsia

Monocytosis, lymphocytosis, thrombocytopenia, nonregenerative anemia, hyperglobulinemia, hypocellular bone marrow, proteinuria, polyclonal or monoclonal gammopathy, nonseptic suppurative polyarthritis, cerebrospinal fluid (CSF) mononuclear pleocytosis

Increased alanine aminotransferase (ALT) and alkaline phosphatase (ALP)

Positive *Ehrlichia* titer, PCR positive

Mycoses, Systemic

CLINICAL FINDINGS

Blastomycosis

Restricted primarily to Mississippi, Ohio, Missouri, Tennessee, and St. Lawrence River valleys plus the southern Great Lakes and the southern Mid-Atlantic states

Sporting breeds predisposed because of greater exposure, males more than females

Anorexia, depression, weight loss, cachexia, fever, mild to severe dyspnea, cyanosis, cough, chylothorax, diffuse lymphadenopathy, papules, plaques and ulcerative nodules, paronychia, chorioretinitis, subretinal granulomas, retinal detachment, lameness from osteomyelitis, splenomegaly

Radiographically, infiltrative bronchointerstitial and
alveolar disease, hilar lymphadenopathy

Histoplasmosis

Restricted primarily to Mississippi, Missouri, and Ohio
River valleys and Mid-Atlantic states

Sporting breeds predisposed because of greater exposure

Common clinical signs include anorexia, fever,
depression, weight loss, cough, dyspnea, diarrhea
(large bowel diarrhea most often, may see protein-
losing enteropathy), hepatosplenomegaly, icterus,
ascites, and lymphadenopathy.

Less common signs include lameness secondary to
osteomyelitis or polyarthritis, chorioretinitis, central
nervous system (CNS) disease, and cutaneous lesions.

Coccidioidomycosis

Primarily southwestern United States, California, Mexico,
Central and South America

Common clinical signs include lameness with swollen
and painful joints and bones, cough, dyspnea,
anorexia, weakness, pleural effusion, and cutaneous
lesions over infected bones.

Less common signs include myocarditis, icterus,
renomegaly, splenomegaly, hepatomegaly, orchitis,
epididymitis, keratitis, iritis, granulomatous uveitis,
glaucoma, seizures, ataxia, and central vestibular
disease.

Cryptococcosis

Found worldwide, more common in southern United
States, most common in cats

Common clinical signs include upper respiratory signs,
unilateral to bilateral nasal discharge, soft masses in
nasal cavity or over bridge of nose, ulcerative skin
lesions, lymphadenopathy, granulomatous
chorioretinitis, and retinal detachment.

Less common signs include fever, lung involvement,
CNS involvement caused by invasion through
cribriform plate, depression, seizures, circling, ataxia,
blindness, head pressing, and paresis.

Aspergillosis

Dogs affected more often than cats

Nasal turbinate destruction, frontal sinus osteomyelitis,
mucoid to hemorrhagic nasal discharge, epistaxis

May lead to masticatory muscle atrophy and CNS disease
by erosion through cribriform plate

In rare cases, disseminates and causes multiple-organ
disease

Pythiosis, Lagenidiosis *(Pythium insidiosum, Lagenidium giganteum)*

Severe, often fatal, chronic gastrointestinal and
cutaneous diseases

Zygomycosis (Multiple Fungi in Class Zygomycetes)

Nasopharyngeal involvement, poorly responsive to
therapy

Polysystemic Protozoal Diseases

CLINICAL FINDINGS

Feline Toxoplasmosis

Acute toxoplasmosis: may induce a self-limiting, small
bowel diarrhea

Disseminated toxoplasmosis: overwhelming intracellular
replication of tachyzoites after primary infection—
depression, anorexia, fever, hypothermia, peritoneal
effusion, icterus, dyspnea, death—coinfection with
feline leukemia virus (FeLV), feline immunodeficiency
virus (FIV), feline infectious peritonitis (FIP), and
others may predispose to disseminated toxoplasmosis.

Chronic toxoplasmosis: anterior or posterior uveitis,
fever, muscle hyperesthesia, weight loss, anorexia,
seizures, ataxia, icterus, diarrhea, pancreatitis

Canine Toxoplasmosis

Respiratory, gastrointestinal, neuromuscular signs: fever,
vomiting, diarrhea, dyspnea, icterus, ataxia, seizures,
tremors, cranial nerve deficits, paresis, paralysis,
myositis, lower motor neuron disease, myocardial
disease, chorioretinitis, anterior uveitis, iridocyclitis,
optic neuritis (ocular lesions less common in dogs
than cats)

Neosporosis

Most common in neonates, but can be seen at any age

Ascending paralysis, hyperextension of hindlimbs,
muscle atrophy, polymyositis, multifocal CNS disease,

myocarditis, dysphagia, ulcerative dermatitis, pneumonia, hepatitis

Babesiosis

Anemia, fever, pale mucous membranes, tachycardia, tachypnea, depression, anorexia, weakness, icterus, petechiae, hepatosplenomegaly, disseminated intravascular coagulation (DIC), metabolic acidosis, renal disease

Cytauxzoonosis

Fever, anorexia, dyspnea (pneumonitis), depression, icterus, pale mucous membranes, death

Hepatozoonosis (*Hepatozoon canis* and *H. americanum*)

Most common in puppies and immunosuppressed dogs, but *H. americanum* can be primary

Fever, weight loss, severe hyperesthesia, anorexia, anemia, depression, oculonasal discharge, bloody diarrhea

Leishmaniasis

Weight loss, normal to increased appetite, polyuria/polydipsia, muscle wasting, depression, vomiting, diarrhea, cough, epistaxis, sneezing, melena, splenomegaly, facial alopecia, rhinitis, dermatitis, icterus, swollen and painful joints, uveitis, conjunctivitis

Dermatologic lesions include hyperkeratosis, scaling, mucocutaneous ulcers, and intradermal nodules on muzzle, ears, and footpads.

American Trypanosomiasis *(Trypanosoma cruzi)*

Acute infection: myocarditis, heart failure—lymphadenopathy, pale mucous membranes, tachycardia, pulse deficits, hepatomegaly, abdominal distension, anorexia, diarrhea, neurologic signs

Chronic infection: those that survive acute infection may present with chronic dilative cardiomyopathy—right-sided heart failure, conductive disturbances, supraventricular arrhythmias.

Rocky Mountain Spotted Fever

CLINICAL FINDINGS
Depression/lethargy
Fever
Anorexia
Myalgia/arthralgia
Lymphadenopathy
Vestibular deficits
Conjunctivitis/scleral congestion/hyphema
Pneumonitis/dyspnea/cough
Abdominal pain
Edema of face and extremities
Epistaxis
Anterior uveitis
Rash/petechiae
Nausea/vomiting
Diarrhea
Vasculitis/thrombocytopenia/disseminated intravascular coagulation (DIC)
Hyperesthesia/spinal cord signs
Seizures
Cardiac arrhythmias
Icterus
Acute renal failure
Coma/stupor
Polyuria/polydipsia

Sepsis and Systemic Inflammatory Response Syndrome (SIRS)

DEFINITIONS
Sepsis: infection-induced systemic inflammation
Severe sepsis: organ dysfunction secondary to sepsis
Septic shock: hypotension secondary to sepsis, not responsive to intravenous (IV) fluid therapy
SIRS: systemic inflammation caused by either infectious or noninfectious processes

NONINFECTIOUS CAUSES OF SIRS
Pancreatitis
Tissue trauma
Heat stroke

Ischemia
Burns
Pansystemic neoplasia

INFECTIOUS CAUSES OF SIRS (SEPSIS)
Peritonitis
Pyometra
Prostatitis
Prostatic abscess
Pyelonephritis
Pneumonia
Pyothorax
Gastroenteritis
Endocarditis
Nosocomial infections (IV catheters, urinary catheters, etc.)

CLINICAL FINDINGS OF SEPSIS AND SIRS
Fever or hypothermia
Tachycardia, tachypnea
Neutrophilia with left shift
Depression
Bounding or diminished pulses
Thrombocytopenia
Hypoalbuminemia, hypoglycemia
Disseminated intravascular coagulation (DIC)
Bilirubinemia
Elevated hepatic enzymes
Azotemia
Oliguria
Lactic acidosis
Hypoxemia
Signs related to underlying condition

Viruses, Canine

COMMON VIRAL AGENTS OF DISEASES OF DOGS
Parvovirus
  May be asymptomatic or fulminant disease
  Anorexia, lethargy, fever, vomiting, hemorrhagic
    diarrhea, myocarditis (rare)
  Worse in very young and parasitized puppies
  Neutropenia, hypoalbuminemia, severe dehydration,
    secondary septicemia

Coronavirus

Diarrhea (infrequently blood in feces), vomiting, anorexia, lethargy, often self-limiting

Rotavirus

Vomiting, diarrhea (rarely bloody), anorexia, typically recover after 5-7 days

Adenovirus Type 1 (Infectious Canine Hepatitis)

Fever, anorexia, lethargy, depression, abdominal pain, pale mucous membranes, tonsillitis, pharyngitis, coughing, hepatomegaly

Severe cases: coagulation abnormalities, petechiae, ecchymosis, DIC, rarely icterus, hepatic encephalopathy

Canine Distemper Virus

See the next section.

Rabies Virus

Variable incubation period, prodromal phase: nervousness, anxiety, paresthesia

Progress to forebrain signs ("furious" form of rabies): irritability, restlessness, pica, photophobia, hyperesthesia progressing to incoordination, seizures, and death

May also progress to "dumb" form: paralysis, lower motor disease, leading to coma, respiratory paralysis, and death

Pseudorabies

Suspected to be result from ingestion of infected raw pork

Neurologic dysfunction: ataxia, abnormal papillary light response, restlessness, trismus, cervical rigidity, ptyalism, tachypnea, excoriation from pruritus of head and neck; most dogs die within 48 hours.

Parainfluenza and Adenovirus Type 2

Hacking cough with gagging, easily elicited with tracheal palpation; cough may be paroxysmal, usually subsides within 7-10 days, and may lead to secondary bacterial or mycoplasmal infection.

Canine Herpesvirus

Abortion, stillbirths; puppies born live progress to crying, hypothermia, soft stools, petechiae, cessation of nursing, and death.

Older puppies develop mild respiratory signs that may emerge later as neurologic disease (ataxia, blindness, central vestibular disease).

Adult dogs: vaginal or preputial hyperemia, hyperplasia of vaginal mucosal lymphoid follicles, submucosal hemorrhage

Canine Oral Papillomavirus

Oral papilloma (warts), may be quite extensive, spontaneously regress

CANINE DISTEMPER VIRUS INFECTION, CLINICAL FINDINGS
General Signs

Fever
Lethargy
Depression
Anorexia
Dehydration

Respiratory Tract

Mucoid to mucopurulent discharge
Bronchopneumonia
- Coughing
- Crackles on auscultation
- Increased bronchovesicular sounds
- Dyspnea
Sneezing

Gastrointestinal Tract

Vomiting
Small bowel diarrhea

Ocular Disease

Mucopurulent ocular discharge
Chorioretinitis, medallion lesions, optic neuritis
Keratoconjunctivitis sicca

Neurologic Disease

Spinal cord lesion: paresis and ataxia
Central vestibular disease: head tilt, nystagmus, other cranial nerve and conscious proprioception deficits
Cerebellar disease: ataxia, head bobbing, hypermetria
Cerebral disease: seizures, blindness
Chorea myoclonus: rhythmic jerking of single muscles or muscle groups

Miscellaneous
Tonsillar enlargement
Pustular dermatosis
Hyperkeratosis of nose and footpads
Enamel hypoplasia

In Utero Infection
Stillbirth
Abortion
"Fading puppy" syndrome in neonatal period
Central nervous system signs at birth

Viruses, Feline

FELINE INFECTIOUS PERITONITIS (FIP, FELINE CORONAVIRUS INFECTION), CLINICAL FINDINGS

Signalment and History
Purebred cats from cattery
Multicat households
< 5 years or >10 years of age
Previous history of mild, self-limiting gastrointestinal or respiratory disease
Anorexia, weight loss, depression
Seizures, nystagmus, ataxia
Acute, fulminant course in cats with effusive FIP
Chronic, intermittent course in cats with noneffusive FIP

Physical Examination Findings
Fever
Weight loss
Abdominal distension/fluid wave
Abdominal mass (focal intestinal granuloma, lymphadenopathy)
Icterus
Muffled heart or lung sounds
Dyspnea secondary to pleural effusion
Hepatomegaly
Chorioretinitis, iridocyclitis
Splenomegaly
Pale mucous membranes with or without petechiae
Multifocal neurologic abnormalities
Irregularly marginated kidneys
Renomegaly

Clinicopathologic Abnormalities

Complete blood count (CBC): nonregenerative anemia, neutrophilia with or without left shift, lymphopenia

Serum chemistry: elevated alkaline phosphatase (ALP) and alanine aminotransferase (ALT), hyperbilirubinemia, hyperglobulinemia (polyclonal, rarely monoclonal gammopathy), azotemia (prerenal or renal)

Urinalysis: proteinuria

Nonseptic, pyogranulomatous exudate in peritoneal cavity, pleural space, and pericardium

Positive coronavirus antibody titer (especially in noneffusive cases)

Cerebrospinal fluid (CSF) tap: increased protein concentration, neutrophilic pleocytosis, coronavirus antibodies

Histopathology: pyogranulomatous inflammation in perivascular locations of tissues

Positive for coronavirus on immunofluorescence or reverse-transcriptase polymerase chain reaction (RT-PCR) testing of abdominal or pleural effusions

FELINE IMMUNODEFICIENCY VIRUS (FIV) INFECTION, CLINICAL FINDINGS

Primary Phase of Infection

Low-grade fever

Lymphadenopathy

Neutropenia

Latent Phase

No clinical signs for months to years

Immunodeficiency Phase

Primary Viral Effects

Nonregenerative anemia, neutropenia, thrombocytopenia

Small bowel diarrhea

Glomerulonephritis

Myeloproliferative disorders

Lymphoma

Renal failure

Anterior uveitis, pars planitis

Behavioral abnormalities

Opportunistic Infectious Agents

Cutaneous: atypical mycobacteriosis, demodicosis, *Notoedres* and *Otodectes* infestation, dermatophytosis, cryptococcosis, cowpox

Gastrointestinal: cryptosporidiosis, coccidiosis, giardiasis, salmonellosis, campylobacteriosis, others

Renal: bacterial infections, FIP, feline leukemia virus (FeLV)

Urinary tract: bacterial infections

Neoplasia: FeLV

Hematologic: *Mycoplasma haemofelis*, FeLV, bartonellosis

Neurologic: toxoplasmosis, cryptococcosis, FIP, FeLV

Ophthalmologic: toxoplasmosis, FIP, cryptococcosis, herpesvirus, bartonellosis

Pneumonia/pneumonitis: bacterial, toxoplasmosis, cryptococcosis

Pyothorax: bacterial

Stomatitis: calicivirus, bacterial, candidiasis, bartonellosis

Upper respiratory: herpesvirus, calicivirus, bacterial, cryptococcosis

FELINE LEUKEMIA VIRUS (FeLV), CLINICAL FINDINGS

General Signs

Anorexia

Weight loss

Depression

Neoplastic

Lymphoma: mediastinal, multicentric, alimentary, renal

Leukemia: lymphocytic, myelogenous, erythroid, megakaryocytic

Myeloproliferative disorders

Fibrosarcoma

Icterus

Prehepatic: immune-mediated red blood cell (RBC) destruction induced by FeLV or secondary infection with *Mycoplasma haemofelis*

Hepatic: hepatic lymphoma, focal liver necrosis, hepatic lipidosis

Posthepatic: alimentary lymphoma

Stomatitis
Bacterial infection
Calicivirus infection

Rhinitis/Pneumonia
Bacteria
Herpesvirus and calicivirus

Renal
Glomerulonephritis
Renal failure
Urinary incontinence: sphincter incompetence or detrusor hyperactivity

Ocular
Lymphoma
Aqueous flare, mass lesions, keratitic precipitates, lens luxations, glaucoma, anterior uveitis

Neurologic
Polyneuropathy or lymphoma
Anisocoria, ataxia, weakness, tetraparesis, paraparesis, behavioral changes, urinary incontinence
Secondary infection with FIP, *Toxoplasma gondii, Cryptococcus neoformans*

In Utero Infection
Abortion, stillbirth, infertility, kitten mortality complex ("fading kitten" syndrome)

Lameness
Neutrophilic polyarthritis secondary to immune complex deposition
Multiple cartilaginous exostoses

OTHER FELINE VIRAL DISEASES
Upper Respiratory Tract Viruses
Herpesvirus type 1: ocular and nasal disease
Calicivirus: ocular, nasal, and oral disease; rarely joint disease

Enteric Viruses
Feline parvovirus (panleukopenia virus): enteritis, panleukopenia, cerebellar hypoplasia, fetal death
Feline coronavirus: mild enteritis, FIP
Rotavirus: rare cause of mild diarrhea
Astrovirus: uncommon cause of persistent watery diarrhea

Torovirus: may be associated with protruding nictitating
  membrane and diarrhea syndrome

Miscellaneous

Cowpox virus: mainly see skin lesions; not seen in North
  America

Hantavirus: zoonotic disease of wild rodents; clinical
  significance in cats not known

Rabies virus

Pseudorabies virus

Feline herpesvirus type 2: possible association with feline
  idiopathic lower urinary tract disease

Joint and Bone Disorders

Arthritis
Bone Disorders

Arthritis

DIFFERENTIAL DIAGNOSIS: INFECTIOUS ARTHRITIS
Septic Arthritis
Bacterial Suppurative Arthritis
Penetrating wounds
- Animal bites

Iatrogenic
- Infection during surgery, arthrocentesis

Trauma (e.g., hit by car)
Hematogenous
- Endocarditis
- Omphalophlebitis
- Pyoderma
- Other foci of infection

Lyme Arthritis
Borrelia burgdorferi
Transmitted by *Ixodes* ticks

Bacterial L-Form Arthritis
Cell wall–deficient bacteria
Causes suppurative arthritis and subcutaneous abscesses
in cats

Mycoplasma Arthritis
Debilitated and immunosuppressed animals
M. gatae, M. felis in cats

Fungal Arthritis (Rare)
Coccidioides immitis
Blastomyces dermatitidis
Filobasidiella (Cryptococcus) neoformans
Sporothrix schenckii
Aspergillus terreus

Rickettsial Arthritis

Rocky Mountain spotted fever (*Rickettsia rickettsii*)
Ehrlichiosis

Protozoal Arthritis

Leishmaniasis *(Leishmania donovani)*
Toxoplasmosis (rare)
Neosporosis *(Neospora caninum)*: polyarthritis,
polymyositis, neurologic disease
Hepatozoonosis: polyarthritis and polymyositis in dog
and cat
Babesiosis (rare, more often causes severe anemia)

Viral Arthritis

Calicivirus infection in cats

Bone Disorders

**DIFFERENTIAL DIAGNOSIS: CONGENITAL, DEVELOPMENTAL,
GENETIC**

Congenital

Hemimelia, phocomelia, amelia: absence of portions or
entire limb (amelia)
Syndactyly: fusion of two or more digits; rarely clinically
significant
Polydactyly: extra digits
Ectrodactyly: third metacarpal and digit missing forming
a cleft (split or "lobster" claw)
Segmented hemiatrophy: limb hypoplasia

Developmental and Genetic

Osteopetrosis: rare; diaphysis remains filled with bone,
marrow does not form, fragile bones
Osteogenesis imperfecta: heritable diseases—fragile bones
Mucopolysaccharidosis: rare lysosomal storage disease—
Siamese cats—causes dwarfism, facial dysmorphism
Dwarfism
• Osteochondrodysplasias
• Pituitary dwarfism
• Congenital hypothyroidism
Retained cartilage cores
Craniomandibular osteopathy (West Highland White
Terrier, Scottish Terrier, Cairn Terrier, Boston Terrier,
other terriers)
Multiple cartilaginous exostoses

DIFFERENTIAL DIAGNOSIS: METABOLIC, NUTRITIONAL, ENDOCRINE, IDIOPATHIC

Metabolic

Nutritional secondary hyperparathyroidism
Lead poisoning

Nutritional

Rickets (hypovitaminosis D)
Renal osteodystrophy
Hypervitaminosis A: causes osteopathy
Hypovitaminosis A: deformed bones secondary to impedance of bone remodeling
Hypervitaminosis D: skeletal demineralization
Zinc-responsive chondrodysplasia
Copper deficiency
Overnutrition of growing dogs

Endocrine

Primary hyperparathyroidism
Humoral hypercalcemia of malignancy
Hyperadrenocorticism
Hypogonadism: delay in physis closure after early gonadectomy
Hepatic osteodystrophy
Anticonvulsant osteodystrophy

Idiopathic

Enostosis (panosteitis)
Metaphyseal osteopathy (hypertrophic osteodystrophy)
Avascular necrosis of femoral head (Legg-Calvé-Perthes disease)
Secondary hypertrophic osteopathy (usually in response to thoracic neoplasia)
Medullary bone infarction
Bone cyst
Aneurysmal bone cyst
Subchondral bone cyst
Fibrous dysplasia
Central giant cell granuloma

Liver and Exocrine Pancreatic Disorders

Cholangitis and Cholangiohepatitis, Feline

COMPARATIVE CLINICAL FINDINGS
Suppurative Cholangitis and Cholangiohepatitis
Middle-aged to older cats
Often depressed and ill
Anorexia (usually)
Jaundice
Neutrophilia
Increased alanine aminotransferase (ALT)
Increased alkaline phosphatase (ALP)
Increased bilirubin
Increased serum and urine bile acids
Hyperechoic liver and bile stasis
Primarily neutrophilic infiltrate
Lesions surround bile ducts
May be associated with pancreatitis and/or inflammatory bowel disease
Respond to antibiotics and choleretics

Lymphocytic Cholangitis

Younger cats
Persians
Polyphagia (±)
Ascites (±)
Lymphadenopathy (±)
Hepatomegaly (±)
Neutrophilia (±)
Lymphopenia (±)
Bile acids (±)
Increased ALT
Increased ALP
Bilirubinemia/bilirubinuria
Hyperglobulinemia
Hyperechoic liver (±)
Primarily lymphocytic infiltrate
Lesions found in portal areas
Variable fibrosis
Pancreatitis (may be present)
Positive response to immunosuppressive corticosteroids

Exocrine Pancreatic Disease

DIFFERENTIAL DIAGNOSIS

Pancreatitis
- Acute
- Chronic

Pancreatic pseudocyst
Pancreatic abscess
Exocrine pancreatic neoplasia
- Pancreatic adenoma
- Pancreatic adenocarcinoma
- Pancreatic sarcoma (spindle cell sarcoma, lymphosarcoma) rare

Nodular hyperplasia
Pancreatic parasites (cats)
- *Eurytrema procyonis* (pancreatic fluke)
- *Amphimerus pseudofelineus* (hepatic fluke)

Pancreatic bladder
- Abnormal extension of pancreatic duct (rare finding in cat)

Hepatic encephalopathy
- Depression
- Ptyalism
Hepatomegaly

Clinicopathologic Findings
Typical findings of cholestasis
- Moderate increase in alanine aminotransferase (ALT)
- Marked increase in alkaline phosphatase (ALP)
- Mild increase in gamma glutamyltransferase (GGT); disproportionately low compared to other feline cholestatic hepatopathies
- Elevated serum bile acids typical

Coagulation test abnormalities (especially in conjunction with acute pancreatitis)

Cytology (Ultrasound-Guided Needle Aspirates) and Histopathology
Reveal clear vacuolation of most hepatocytes, nonzonal in distribution; typically with absence of inflammatory cells

Hepatobiliary Disease

CLINICAL AND PHYSICAL FINDINGS
General Clinical Features
Depression
Anorexia
Lethargy
Weight loss
Poor haircoat, insufficient grooming
Nausea, vomiting
Diarrhea
Dehydration
Small body stature

Signs Specific but Not Pathognomonic for Hepatic Disease
Icterus
Bilirubinuria
Acholic feces
Organomegaly
Ascites

CLINICAL FINDINGS OF EXOCRINE PANCREATIC INSUFFICIENCY
Most often seen in young to middle-aged dogs; German Shepherds are predisposed.
Chronic weight loss
Ravenous appetite
Coprophagia
Pica
Change in fecal character
- Voluminous
- Soft
- Watery
- May be normal
Poor haircoat quality
Coagulation disorder (caused by malabsorption of vitamin K, rare)

Gallbladder and Extrahepatic Biliary Disease

DIFFERENTIAL DIAGNOSIS
Obstructive Disease
Extrahepatic biliary obstruction
- Pancreatitis (most common etiology in dog)
- Biliary neoplasia
- Cholangitis
- Pancreatic neoplasia
Cholelithiasis
Gallbladder mucocele

Nonobstructive Disease
Cholecystitis
- Bacterial cholecystitis (ascending infection— *Escherichia coli* most common)
- Necrotizing cholecystitis
- Emphysematous cholecystitis (*E. coli, Clostridium perfringens*)
Cholelithiasis (does not always cause obstruction)
Parasites (mainly seen in cats)
- *Platynosomum fastosum* (a fluke)
Tropical climates (seen in cats that eat lizards or toads)
- *Amphimerus pseudofelineus*
- *Metorchis conjunctus*
- *Eurytrema procyonis*

Neoplasia
Bile duct carcinoma

Caroli's Disease
Dilatation of intrahepatic and extrahepatic bile ducts

Gallbladder Rupture
Necrotizing cholecystitis
Obstruction
Iatrogenic
Blunt abdominal trauma

CLINICAL FINDINGS OF GALLBLADDER AND BILIARY DISEASE
Clinical Signs
Vomiting
Icterus
Anorexia
Fever
Abdominal pain
Depression
Weight loss
Ascites

Clinicopathologic Findings
Hyperbilirubinemia
Elevated alkaline phosphatase (ALP) levels
Elevated gamma glutamyltransferase (GGT) levels
Elevated serum bile acids
Elevated alanine aminotransferase (ALT) levels

Radiographic Findings
Hepatomegaly
Mass effect in area of gallbladder
Gas shadow in area of gallbladder
Choleliths radiopaque if they contain calcium (50% may
    not be seen on radiographs)

Ultrasonographic Signs
Dilated and tortuous bile ducts
Gallbladder distension
Cholelith visible
Pancreatic mass identified
Stellate appearance to contents of gallbladder
    (characteristic of a gallbladder mucocele)

Hepatic Encephalopathy

CLINICAL FINDINGS
General Systemic Clinical Signs
Anorexia
Depression
Weight loss
Lethargy
Nausea
Fever
Ptyalism
Intermittent vomiting
Diarrhea

Central Nervous System Clinical Signs
Tremors
Ataxia
Personality change (often toward aggression)
Dementia
Head pressing
Circling
Hysteria
Cortical blindness
Seizures

Hepatic Lipidosis, Feline

CLINICAL FINDINGS
Historical Findings
Obesity
Recent anorexia and rapid weight loss
- Concurrent disease that causes anorexia (pancreatitis,
  diabetes mellitus, inflammatory hepatobiliary disease,
  inflammatory bowel disease, feline infectious
  peritonitis, chronic renal failure, neoplasia,
  cardiomyopathy, neurologic disease, etc.)
- Stressful event
- Abrupt diet change
Typically indoor cats

Physical Findings
Jaundice
Vomiting
Dehydration

Hepatic encephalopathy
- Behavioral changes (aggression, dementia, hysteria)
- Circling
- Ataxia
- Staggering
- Pacing
- Head pressing
- Cortical blindness
- Ptyalism
- Tremors/seizures
- Coma

Coagulopathies

Polydipsia/polyuria

CAUSES OF ELEVATED SERUM HEPATOBILIARY ENZYMES
Primary Hepatic Disease

Drug Induction
Corticosteroids (dogs)
Anticonvulsants (phenobarbital, phenytoin, primidone)

Endocrinopathies
Hyperadrenocorticism (dogs)
Hypothyroidism (dogs)
Hyperthyroidism (cats)
Diabetes mellitus

Bone Disorders
Growing animals
Osteosarcoma
Osteomyelitis

Neoplasia
Adenocarcinomas (pancreatic, intestinal, adrenocortical, mammary)
Sarcomas (hemangiosarcoma, leiomyosarcoma)
Hepatic metastasis

Muscle Injury
Acute muscle necrosis/trauma
Myopathies
Malignant hyperthermia

Hypoxia/Hypotension
Septic shock
Surgery
Congestive heart failure
Hypoadrenocorticism

Circulatory shock
Severe acute blood loss
Hypotensive crisis
Status epilepticus

Miscellaneous Causes
Systemic infections
Pregnancy (cats—increased placental alkaline
  phosphatase)
Colostrum-fed neonates (dogs)

DIFFERENTIAL DIAGNOSIS, DOGS
Inflammation
Chronic hepatitis complex
- Copper accumulation—Bedlington Terrier, Airedale
  Terrier, Bull Terrier, Bulldog, Cocker Spaniel, Collie,
  Dachshund, Dalmatian, Doberman Pinscher, German
  Shepherd, Golden Retriever, Keeshond, Kerry Blue
  Terrier, Labrador Retriever, Norwich Terrier, Old
  English Sheepdog, Pekingese, Poodle, Samoyed,
  Schnauzer, Skye Terrier, West Highland White Terrier,
  Wire Fox Terrier
- Drug induced: trimethoprim-sulfa, phenobarbital,
  diethylcarbamazine, oxibendazole, many others
- Familial hepatitis—Doberman Pinscher, West
  Highland White Terrier, Dalmatian, Skye Terrier,
  Cocker Spaniel
Fibrosis and cirrhosis
Infectious agents: leptospirosis, canine adenovirus type 2
  infection, bacterial hepatitis, histoplasmosis, Rocky
  Mountain spotted fever, ehrlichiosis, babesiosis
Cholangiohepatitis
Granulomatous hepatitis
- *Rhodococcus, Borrelia, Bartonella, Histoplasma,
  Coccidioidomyces, Hepatozoon, Heterobilharzia* spp.
Acidophil cell hepatitis
Lobular dissecting hepatitis
Hepatic abscess

Acute Toxic or Drug-Induced Hepatopathy

Vacuolar Hepatopathy

Metabolic Liver Disease
Amyloidosis
Hyperlipidemia
Lysosomal storage disease

Vascular Hepatic Disease
Congenital portosystemic venous anomaly
Intrahepatic portal vein hypoplasia
Intrahepatic arteriovenous fistula

Biliary Tract Disease

Neoplasia
Primary: hepatocellular carcinoma, hepatocellular
  adenoma, hepatic hemangiosarcoma, biliary
  carcinoma
Other hepatic tumors: leiomyosarcoma, liposarcoma,
  myxosarcoma, fibrosarcoma, biliary adenoma, hepatic
  carcinoid
Hemolymphatic: lymphosarcoma, mast cell tumor,
  plasma cell tumor
Metastatic neoplasia

Hepatic or Biliary Cysts

DIFFERENTIAL DIAGNOSIS, CATS
Hepatic Lipidosis

Inflammatory Hepatobiliary Disease
Cholangitis/cholangiohepatitis complex
  • Suppurative cholangitis, cholangiohepatitis
  • Lymphocytic cholangitis
Chronic cholangiohepatitis (later stage of acute
  cholangiohepatitis)
Sclerosing cholangitis
Lymphocytic portal hepatitis
Feline infectious peritonitis (FIP)

Toxic Hepatopathy
Antimicrobials (trimethoprim-sulfa, tetracycline)
Anticonvulsants (phenobarbital)
Diazepam
Methimazole
Griseofulvin
Ketoconazole
Pine oils (cleaning agents)
Amanita phalloides (death cap mushroom)
Natural or herbal remedies
Many others

Portosystemic Venous Anomaly

Lipoprotein Lipase Deficiency

Neoplasia

Primary Hepatic Neoplasia
Biliary carcinoma
Hepatocellular carcinoma
Hepatic hemangiosarcoma
Bilary cystadenoma
Myelolipoma
Hepatic carcinoid

Hemolymphatic Neoplasia
Lymphosarcoma
Mast cell tumor
Plasma cell tumor

Metastatic Neoplasia

Hepatomegaly and Microhepatica

DIFFERENTIAL DIAGNOSIS

Generalized Hepatomegaly
Acute toxic hepatopathy
Infiltrative hepatic disease
- Neoplasia: primary or metastatic
- Chronic hepatitis complex (dog)
- Cholangiohepatitis (cat)
- Extramedullary hematopoiesis
- Mononuclear-phagocytic cell hyperplasia
- Amyloidosis (rare)
Passive congestion
- Right-sided heart failure
- Pericardial disease (dog)
- Caval syndrome (dog)
- Caudal vena cava obstruction (dog)
- Budd-Chiari syndrome (rare)
Hepatocellular hypertrophy
- Hepatic lipidosis
- Steroid hepatopathy
- Anticonvulsant drug therapy
Acute extrahepatic bile duct obstruction

Focal Hepatomegaly
Neoplasia: primary or metastatic
Nodular hyperplasia
Chronic hepatic disease with fibrosis and nodular regeneration

Hepatic abscess
Hepatic cyst

Microhepatica
Decreased hepatic mass
- Chronic hepatic disease with progressive loss of hepatocytes

Decreased portal blood flow with hepatocellular atrophy
- Congenital portosystemic shunt
- Intrahepatic portal vein hypoplasia
- Chronic portal vein thrombosis

Hypovolemia
- Hypoadrenocorticism
- Shock

Hyperlipidemia

DIFFERENTIAL DIAGNOSIS
Primary
Idiopathic hyperlipidemia of Miniature Schnauzers
Feline familial hyperchylomicronemia
Idiopathic hypercholesterolemia (rare—Doberman Pinscher, Rottweiler)

Secondary
Endocrine
- Hypothyroidism
- Diabetes mellitus
- Hyperadrenocorticism

Nephrotic syndrome
Cholestasis
Drug induced
- Glucocorticoids
- Megesterol acetate

CLINICAL FINDINGS
Severe Hyperlipidemia
Intermittent gastrointestinal signs
- Vomiting
- Diarrhea
- Abdominal discomfort

Pancreatitis
Lipemia retinalis
Cutaneous xanthomas

Peripheral nerve paralysis
Behavioral changes

Severe Hypercholesterolemia
Arcus lipoides corneae
Lipemia retinalis
Atherosclerosis

Pancreatitis

CLINICAL FINDINGS OF ACUTE PANCREATITIS
Dogs
Mild Acute Pancreatitis
Depression
Anorexia
Nausea, vomiting, diarrhea
Ptyalism
Mild right cranial abdominal pain
Fever, dehydration, weakness

Moderate to Severe Acute Pancreatitis
Depression
Anorexia
Vomiting
Right cranial abdominal pain
Hematemesis, hematochezia, melena
Jaundice
Respiratory distress
Shock, fever, dehydration
Hyperemic mucous membranes
Tachycardia, tachypnea
Abdominal effusion
Mass effect in region of pancreas
Petechiae, ecchymoses
Cardiac arrhythmia
Glossitis, glossal slough
Extrahepatic biliary obstruction

Cats
Signs tend to be more subclinical and nonspecific.
May be associated with inflammatory bowel disease
May be component of multisystemic disease such as
    toxoplasmosis
Lethargy, anorexia, vomiting, dehydration, weight loss,
    jaundice, hypothermia

May present as acute necrotizing or acute suppurative
form

PREDISPOSING FACTORS
Nutritional
Obesity
High-fat diet
After ingestion of large, fatty meal

Hyperlipoproteinemia
Idiopathic in Miniature Schnauzers

Drugs
Chemotherapeutic agents
- L-Asparaginase
- Azathioprine
- Others
Organophosphates
Corticosteroids (controversial)

Ischemia
Hypovolemia
Associated with disseminated intravascular coagulation
(DIC)
Vasoactive amine–induced vasoconstriction

Duodenal reflex
Increased intraluminal pressure during severe vomiting

Other
Cholangitis
Infection (toxoplasmosis, feline infectious peritonitis)
Abdominal trauma
Hypercalcemia
Hyperadrenocorticism (possibly)

Portosystemic Shunt, Congenital

CLINICAL FINDINGS
Signalment
Young animal, male or female, often purebred

History
Neurologic signs (dementia, circling, personality change,
head pressing, wall hugging, seizures)
Vomiting

Diarrhea
Ptyalism (especially cats)
Worsening of signs after eating
Improvement of signs with antimicrobial therapy
Prolonged recovery from anesthesia
Recurrent urate urolithiasis in breeds other than
    Dalmatian and English Bulldog

Physical Examination
Poor haircoat
Small stature
Cystic calculi
Cryptorchidism
Bilateral renomegaly
Copper-colored irises in non-Asian cat breeds
Other congenital anomalies

Vacuolar Hepatopathy, Canine

DIFFERENTIAL DIAGNOSIS
Hyperadrenocorticism
- Pituitary dependent
- Adrenal dependent
- Iatrogenic (glucocorticoid therapy)
Pancreatitis
- Chronic
Severe hypothyroidism
Chronic stress
- Illness of more than 4 months
Severe dental disease
- Oral infection
Disorders affecting lipid metabolism
- Diabetes mellitus
- Idiopathic hyperlipidemia
Neoplasia
- Lymphoma
Congestive heart failure
Abnormal sex hormone production
Inflammatory bowel disease
- Chronic, lymphoplasmacytic, eosinophilic
Hepatocutaneous syndrome

Neoplasia

Chemotherapeutic Agent Toxicity

Most severely affects tissues with a growth fraction that approaches that of tumor cells.

CLINICAL FINDINGS

Myelosuppression

Neutropenia: short-lived cells; nadir is 5-10 days postchemotherapy.

Thrombocytopenia: nadir is 7-14 days postchemotherapy.

Anemia: erythrocytes live longer; rarely clinically significant.

Gastrointestinal Toxicity

Nausea, vomiting

Diarrhea

Inappetence

Anorexia

Cardiotoxicity

Doxorubicin therapy

Most likely after cumulative dose of 180 mg/m^2

Nephrotoxicity

Cisplatin

Limit use of cisplatin in cases of preexisting renal disease.

Urothelial Toxicity
Sterile hemorrhagic cystitis
Cyclophosphamide, ifosfamide

Extravasation
Doxorubicin: severe local reaction leading to slough
Vincristine: usually minor tissue damage

Hypersensitivity
Doxorubicin: caused by histamine release from mast
cells; prevented by slow administration
L-Asparaginase: less likely if given subcutaneously rather
than intravenously
Etoposide, paclitaxel: caused by carrier solutions for
these agents

Alopecia
Less of a problem in dogs and cats than in people
Worse in breeds that have hair (e.g., Poodles, terriers,
Old English Sheepdogs) than in dogs with fur
Loss of "feathers" (e.g., Golden Retrievers)
Loss of whiskers in cats

Neurologic Toxicity
Fatal neurotoxicity in cats with topical or systemic
administration of 5-fluorouracil

Respiratory Toxicity
Fatal, acute pulmonary edema in cats with cisplatin
therapy

Corticosteroid Therapy

**ADVERSE EFFECTS ASSOCIATED WITH GLUCOCORTICOID
ADMINISTRATION**
Polyuria/polydipsia
Polyphagia
Increased alkaline phosphatase (ALP) levels
Increased gamma glutamyltransferase (GGT) levels
Panting
Insomnia, agitation, behavioral changes
Immunosuppression
- Secondary infection
- Recrudescence of latent infection
- Worsening of existing infection
- Demodicosis

Vacuolar hepatopathy
Iatrogenic hyperadrenocorticism
Adrenocorticoid deficiency with rapid withdrawal after
    sustained use
Alopecia
Calcinosis cutis
Comedones
Skin thinning
Proteinuria
Muscle atrophy/muscle wasting
Myotonia/myopathy
Delayed wound healing
Colonic perforation
Gastrointestinal ulceration
Insulin resistance
Diabetes mellitus
Hyperlipidemia
Abortion
Growth suppression
Hypercoagulable state
Ligament and tendon rupture
Psychosis/behavior change
Lowered seizure threshold

Histiocytic Disease

CLASSIFICATION, DOGS
May be difficult to differentiate from lymphoproliferative,
granulomatous, or reactive inflammatory disease by histopathology alone.

Cutaneous Histiocytoma
Benign, usually solitary lesion
Typically young dogs
Often spontaneously regress

Langerhans' Cell Histiocytoma
Rare, rapidly metastatic, cutaneous infiltration by
    histiocytes

Cutaneous Histiocytosis
Single or multiple lesions
May spontaneously regress
May respond to immunosuppressive drugs

Systemic Histiocytosis

Familial disease of Bernese Mountain Dogs, rarely other breeds

Similar lesions to cutaneous histiocytosis, but may also affect mucous membranes, lymphoid organs, lung, bone marrow, and other organ systems

Progressive, requires immunosuppressive therapy

Histiocytic Sarcoma

Bernese Mountain Dog, Rottweiler, Flat-Coated Retriever, Golden Retriever, rarely other breeds

Histiocytic sarcoma usually begins as a localized lesion in spleen, lymph nodes, lung, bone marrow, skin and subcutis, brain, and periarticular tissue of appendicular joints.

- Rapidly disseminates to multiple organs

Malignant Histiocytosis

Bernese Mountain Dog, Rottweiler, Flat-Coated Retriever, Golden Retriever, rarely other breeds

Multisystemic, rapidly progressive disease of multiple organs

CLASSIFICATION, CATS

Feline Progressive Histiocytosis

Rare, usually see multiple skin nodules, papules, plaques

Head, lower extremities, trunk

Poor long-term prognosis

Feline Histiocytic Sarcoma

Poorly demarcated tumors of subcutis or spleen

Poor prognosis

Lymphoma

COMMON DIFFERENTIAL DIAGNOSES

Generalized Lymphadenopathy

Disseminated infections
- Bacterial, fungal, rickettsial, parasitic, viral

Immune-mediated disease
- Systemic lupus erythematosus (SLE), polyarthritis, vasculitis, dermatopathy

Other hematopoietic tumors
- Leukemia, multiple myeloma, malignant or systemic histiocytosis

Neoplasia metastatic to lymph nodes
Benign reactive hyperplastic syndromes in cats

Alimentary Disease

Inflammatory bowel diseases
- Lymphocytic/plasmacytic, eosinophilic enteritis

Nonlymphoid intestinal neoplasia
Granulomatous enteritis
Granulated round cell tumors in cats
Gastrointestinal mast cell neoplasia in cats

Cutaneous Disease

Infectious dermatitis (deep pyoderma, fungal dermatitis)
Immune-mediated dermatitis (e.g., pemphigus foliaceus)
Other cutaneous neoplasms

Mediastinal Disease

Thymoma
Chemodectoma (heart base tumor)
Ectopic thyroid neoplasia
Pulmonary lymphomatoid granulomatosis
Granulomatous disease (e.g., hilar lymphadenopathy
with blastomycosis)

Paraneoplastic Syndromes

CLASSIFICATION

General

Cancer anorexia, cachexia
Fever

Hematologic

Anemia
- Anemia of chronic disease
- Immune-mediated hemolytic anemia
- Blood loss anemia
- Microangiopathic hemolytic anemia

Polycythemia (rare)
- Associated with renal neoplasia, nasal fibrosarcoma,
bronchial carcinoma, cecal leiomyosarcoma

Leukocytosis
- Neutrophilic
- Eosinophilic

Thrombocytopenia
- Increased consumption

- Decreased production (bone marrow neoplasia)
- Increased destruction (immune-mediated thrombocytopenia)

Thrombocytosis

Thrombocyte hyperaggregability

Pancytopenia

Coagulation disorders

- Disseminated intravascular coagulation (DIC)
- Coagulation-activating substances produced by tumor

Hyperproteinemia

Endocrine
Hypercalcemia of malignancy

Hypoglycemia

Syndrome of inappropriate antidiuretic hormone (ADH) secretion

- Hyponatremia, serum
- Hypoosmolality, urine
- Hyperosmolality

Gastrointestinal
Gastroduodenal ulceration

- Mast cell tumors, gastrinoma

Renal
Glomerulonephritis

Hypercalcemic nephropathy

Cutaneous
Superficial necrolytic dermatitis

Nodular dermatofibrosis

Neuromuscular
Myasthenia gravis

- Dogs with thymoma

Peripheral neuropathy

- Multiple myeloma, lymphoma, various carcinomas and sarcomas

Hypertrophic Osteodystrophy
Space-occupying mass in thorax or rarely abdomen

Sarcomas

CLASSIFICATION OF SOFT TISSUE SARCOMAS
Fibrosarcoma
Undifferentiated sarcoma
Hemangiosarcoma
Hemangiopericytoma
Leiomyosarcoma
Malignant fibrous histiocytoma
Schwannoma
Neurofibrosarcoma
Synovial sarcoma
Rhabdomyosarcoma
Liposarcoma
Vaccine-associated fibrosarcoma (cats)

CLINICAL FINDINGS FOR HEMANGIOSARCOMA
Older dogs and cats
Many potential sites of origin
- Spleen
- Right atrium
- Subcutis
- Pericardium
- Liver
- Muscle
- Lung
- Skin
- Bone
- Kidney
- Central nervous system
- Peritoneum
- Oral cavity

Hemoabdomen
Pericardial effusion
Cardiac tamponade
Sudden death
Anorexia, vomiting
Lethargy
Right-sided heart failure
Muffled heart sounds
Arrhythmias
Neurologic signs

Thyroid Neoplasms

CLASSIFICATION AND CLINICAL FINDINGS
  Cats
    Hyperthyroidism: functional thyroid tumors
    • Thyroid adenoma
    • Thyroid adenocarcinoma

  Dogs
    Nonfunctional tumors (90%)
    Thyroid adenoma
    Thyroid adenocarcinoma
    • Swelling or mass in neck
    • Dyspnea
    • Cough
    • Lethargy
    • Dysphagia
    • Regurgitation
    • Anorexia
    • Weight loss
    • Horner's syndrome
    • Change in bark
    • Facial edema
    Functional tumors (10%)
    Thyroid adenoma
    Thyroid adenocarcinoma
    • Swelling or mass in neck
    • Polyphagia/weight
    • Hyperactivity
    • Polyuria/polydipsia
    • Panting
    • Change in behavior

Tumors

BONE AND JOINT TUMORS, CLASSIFICATION
  Canine osteosarcoma
    Appendicular
    Skull
    Scapular
    Pelvic
    Ribs
    Vertebral
    Nasal and paranasal

Chondrosarcoma
Fibrosarcoma
Hemangiosarcoma
Multilobular osteochondrosarcoma
Osteoma
Canine multiple cartilaginous exostoses
Feline osteosarcoma
Feline multiple cartilaginous exostoses
Metastatic bone tumors
    Transitional cell carcinoma
    Prostatic adenocarcinoma
    Mammary carcinoma
    Thyroid carcinoma
    Pulmonary carcinoma
    Nasal carcinoma
    Apocrine gland, anal sac adenocarcinoma
    Renal tumors
    Others
Primary joint tumors
    Synovial cell sarcoma
    Histiocytic sarcoma
    Malignant fibrous histiocytoma
    Synovial myxoma
    Myxosarcoma
    Osteosarcoma
    Fibrosarcoma
    Chondrosarcoma
    Hemangiosarcoma
    Liposarcoma
    Rhabdomyosarcoma
    Undifferentiated sarcoma

HEMATOPOIETIC TUMORS, CLASSIFICATION

Lymphoma

Feline

    Alimentary
    Multicentric
    Mediastinal/thymic
    Nasal
    Renal
    Other
    Feline leukemia virus (FeLV) associated

Canine

    Multicentric
    Others (alimentary, mediastinal, cutaneous)

Lymphoid Leukemia
Acute lymphoblastic leukemia (in cats, often associated
with FeLV infection)
Chronic lymphocytic leukemia

Nonlymphoid Leukemias and Myeloproliferative Disorders
Acute myelogenous leukemia (myeloblastic)
Acute myelomonocytic leukemia
(myeloblasts/monoblasts)
Acute monocytic leukemia (monoblasts)
Acute megakaryoblastic leukemia (megakaryoblasts)
Erythroleukemia (erythroblasts)

Chronic Myeloproliferative Disorders
Chronic myelogenous leukemia (neutrophils, late
precursors)
Primary thrombocythemia (platelets)
Basophilic leukemia (basophils and precursors)
Eosinophic leukemia (eosinophils and precursors)
Polycythemia vera (erythrocytes)

Plasma Cell Neoplasms
Multiple myeloma
Solitary plasmacytoma

MAST CELL TUMOR (MCT) DISEASE, CLINICAL FINDINGS
Clinical Appearance and Location of MCTs
Extremely variable in appearance
Soft, fluctuant, firm, discrete, diffuse, small, large,
solitary, multiple, haired, hairless, dermal, or
subcutaneous
Erythema, bruising, ulceration
On trunk most often; also perineum, extremities, head,
neck
Rarely oral cavity, nasal cavity, larynx, conjunctiva

Systemic Signs of Disseminated Mastocytosis
Gastrointestinal ulceration
Abdominal discomfort
Vomiting
Melena
Hypotension
Coagulation abnormalities
Acute or chronic blood loss anemia

ORAL CAVITY TUMORS, DIFFERENTIAL DIAGNOSIS
Malignant Neoplasms
Melanoma
Squamous cell carcinoma
Fibrosarcoma

Benign Neoplasms
Epulides
- Fibromatous
- Ossifying
- Acanthomatous (squamous): may be invasive, but does not metastasize

Papillomas: self-limiting
Fibroma
Lipoma
Chondroma
Osteoma
Hemangioma
Hemangiopericytoma
Histiocytoma

SKIN AND SUBCUTANEOUS TUMORS
Epithelial Tumors
Sebaceous gland adenoma/adenocarcinoma
Squamous cell carcinoma
- Canine cutaneous squamous cell carcinoma
- Canine nasal planum squamous cell carcinoma
- Canine digital squamous cell carcinoma
- Feline cutaneous squamous cell carcinoma
- Feline multicentric squamous cell carcinoma in situ (Bowen's disease)

Trichoepithelioma
Intracutaneous cornifying epithelioma
Basal cell tumors
- Benign tumors
- Basal carcinoma

Trichoblastoma
Pilomatricoma
Papilloma
Perianal gland tumors (hepatoid gland tumors)
Sweat gland tumors (apocrine gland tumors)
Ceruminous gland tumors
Anal sac, apocrine gland tumors

Round Cell Tumors
Lymphoma
MCT
Histiocytoma
Transmissible venereal tumor (TVT)
Plasmacytoma

Melanocytic Tumors
Melanoma
- Benign (typically melanomas of haired skin and eyelids)
- Malignant (typically those of digit or mucocutaneous junctions)

UROGENITAL TUMORS, CLASSIFICATION
Kidney
Lymphoma (most common renal tumor in cats)
Primary renal carcinoma, adenocarcinoma
Cystadenocarcinoma with concurrent nodular dermatofibrosis in German Shepherds
Tumors of embryonic origin

Urinary Bladder
Older female dogs, West Highland White Terrier, Scottish Terriers, Beagles, Dachshunds, Shetland Sheepdogs
Transitional cell carcinoma
Squamous cell carcinoma
Leiomyosarcoma
Leiomyoma
Rhabdomyosarcoma
Metastatic neoplasia
- Hemangiosarcoma
- Lymphoma
- Extension of prostate neoplasia

Prostate
Prostatic adenocarcinoma
Transitional cell carcinoma

Penis and Prepuce
Prepuce affected by tumors of haired skin seen elsewhere
Penile
- Transmissible venereal tumor
- Others

Testicular Neoplasia
Testicle
Sertoli cell tumor

Leydig cell (interstitial) tumor
Seminoma

Vagina and Vulva
Leiomyoma
Fibroleiomyoma
Fibroma
Polyps
Lipoma
Leiomyosarcoma
Transmissible venereal tumor (TVT)

Uterus
Leiomyoma
Leiomyosarcoma
Uterine adenocarcinoma

Ovary
Epithelial Tumors
Papillary adenoma
Cystadenoma
Papillary adenocarcinoma
Undifferentiated adenocarcinoma

Germ Cell Tumors
Dysgerminoma
Teratoma
Teratocarcinoma

Sex-Cord Stromal Tumors
Granulosa cell tumor
Benign thecoma
Benign luteoma

Mammary Gland
Fibroadenoma
Solid carcinomas
Tubular adenocarcinoma
Sarcoma
Inflammatory carcinomas
Feline mammary adenocarcinomas

Neurologic and Neuromuscular Disorders

Brain Disease, Congenital or Hereditary

DIFFERENTIAL DIAGNOSIS
  Congenital Malformations
    Failure of normal closure of neural tube: vary in severity
      from clinically inapparent (agenesis of corpus
      callosum) to severe (anencephaly)
    Lissencephaly: failure of normal migration of neurons in
      development of cerebral cortex; leads to abnormal
      appearance of sulci and gyri (most often seen in
      Lhasa Apso)
    Cerebellar hypoplasia: seen most often in cats after in
      utero panleukopenia infection; rarely seen with
      parvovirus infection of developing cerebellum in
      dogs; may be isolated malformation without infection
    Chiari-like malformations: protrusion of cerebellar
      vermis through foramen magnum (Cavalier King
      Charles Spaniel, other dog breeds)
    Hydrocephalus: congenital hydrocephalus seen most
      often in toy and brachycephalic breeds; suggests

hereditary basis; often congenital stenosis or aplasia
of mesencephalic aqueducts

Inborn errors of metabolism (hereditary): young,
purebred animals with diffuse, symmetric signs of
brain disease

- Organic acidurias
- Spongiform encephalopathies: may be hereditary or
acquired (transmissible) disease
- Polioencephalopathies: metabolic defects that affect
gray matter
- Neuroaxonal dystrophy: spheroids causing swelling
within axons
- Leukoencephalopathies: disorders of myelin; affect
white matter; often affect cerebellum and long tracts
leading to tremors and dysmetria
- Lysosomal storage diseases: accumulation of
metabolic products in lysosomes
- Ceroid lipofuscinosis: accumulation of proteins in
lysosomes

Movement Disorders

Hereditary cerebellar hypoplasia

Multisystem degeneration: diseases of cerebellum and
basal ganglia—progressive neuronal abiotrophy of
Kerry Blue Terriers and Chinese Crested dogs

Dyskinesis and dystonias

Paroxysmal dyskinesias ("Scotty cramp" or idiopathic
cerebellitis)—Scottish Terriers

Cognitive Dysfunction

CLINICAL FINDINGS

Disorientation

Sleep/wake cycle alterations

House soiling problems

Change in activity levels

- Increased
- Stereotypic
- Decreased

Agitation

Anxiety

Altered responsiveness to stimuli

- Heightened
- Reduced

Changes in appetite
- Increased
- Decreased

Decreased ability to perform learned tasks

Changes in interaction with owners

Cranial Nerve (CN) Deficits

CLINICAL FINDINGS

CN I (Olfactory)
Loss of ability to smell

CN II (Optic)
Loss of vision, dilated pupil, loss of papillary light reflex (direct and consensual)

CN III (Oculomotor)
Loss of papillary light reflex on affected side (even if light shone in opposite eye), dilated pupil, ventrolateral strabismus

CN IV (Troclear)
Slight dorsomedial eye rotation

CN V (Trigeminal)
Atrophy of temporalis and masseter muscles, loss of jaw tone and strength, dropped jaw (if bilateral), analgesia of innervated areas

CN VI (Abducens)
Medial strabismus, impaired lateral gaze, poor retraction of globe

CN VII (Facial)
Lip, eyelid, and ear droop; loss of ability to blink; loss of ability to retract lip; possibly decreased tear production

CN VIII (Vestibulocochlear)
Ataxia, head tilt, nystagmus, deafness

CN IX (Glossopharyngeal)
Loss of gag reflex, dysphagia

CN X (Vagus)
Loss of gag reflex, laryngeal paralysis, dysphagia

CN XI (Accessory)
Atrophy of trapezius, sternocephalicus, and
brachiocephalicus muscles

CN XII (Hypoglossal)
Loss of tongue strength

Head Tilt

DIFFERENTIAL DIAGNOSIS
Peripheral Vestibular Disease
Otitis media/interna
Feline idiopathic vestibular disease
Geriatric canine vestibular disease
Feline nasopharyngeal polyps
Middle ear tumor
• Ceruminous gland adenocarcinoma
• Squamous cell carcinoma
Trauma
Aminoglycoside ototoxicity
Hypothyroidism (possibly)

Central Vestibular Disease
Trauma/hemorrhage
Infectious inflammatory disease
• Rocky Mountain spotted fever
• Feline infectious peritonitis (fiP)
• Others
Granulomatous meningoencephalitis
Neoplasia
Vascular infarct
Thiamine deficiency
Metronidazole toxicity

Inflammatory Disease of the Nervous System

DIFFERENTIAL DIAGNOSIS
Steroid-responsive suppurative meningitis
Meningeal vasculitis (Beagle, Boxer, Bernese Mountain Dog,
German Shorthaired Pointer)
Granulomatous meningoencephalitis
• Idiopathic inflammatory brain disease of dogs

Pug meningoencephalitis
- Necrotizing meningoencephalitis of cerebral cortex

Feline polioencephalomyelitis
- Young cats, progressive course

Feline immunodeficiency virus (FIV) encephalopathy

Bacterial meningitis and myelitis
- *Staphylococcus aureus*
- *Staphylococcus epidermidis*
- *Staphylococcus albus*
- *Pasteurella multocida*
- *Actinomyces*
- *Nocardia*
- Others

Canine distemper virus

Rabies

Feline infectious peritonitis (FIP)

Toxoplasmosis

Neosporosis

Borreliosis

Mycotic infections
- *Cryptococcus neoformans*
- Other disseminated systemic mycoses

Rickettsial diseases
- Rocky Mountain spotted fever
- Ehrlichiosis

Parasitic meningitis, myelitis, encephalitis
- Aberrant parasite migration

Intracranial Neoplasms

DIFFERENTIAL DIAGNOSIS

Meningioma

Benign tumor of cells of meninges

Neuroepithelial Tumors (Gliomas)

Astrocytomas

Oligodendrogliomas

Choroid plexus tumors (choroid plexus papilloma,
ependymal tumor)

Central Nervous System (CNS) Lymphoma

Primary: neoplasia of native CNS lymphocytes

Secondary: metastasis of systemic lymphoma

Metastatic Neoplasia to CNS
 Local invasion: nasal adenocarcinoma
 Hematogenous spread: melanoma, hemangiosarcoma,
 lymphosarcoma
 Many other neoplasms may metastasize to CNS.

Pituitary Tumors
 Functional tumors of pars distalis or pars intermedius: cause
 pituitary-dependent hyperadrenocorticism; generally
 cause little damage to surrounding tissue
 Pituitary macrotumor

Myasthenia Gravis

Congenital myasthenia gravis: Inherited deficiency of acetylcholine
receptors at presynaptic membranes of skeletal muscle.
Acquired myasthenia gravis: Antibodies made against nicotinic
acetylcholine receptors of skeletal muscle.

CLINICAL FINDINGS
 Appendicular muscle weakness
 • Worsens with exercise
 • Improves with rest
 Mentation, postural reactions, reflexes normal
 Megaesophagus
 • Salivation
 • Regurgitation
 Dysphagia
 Hoarse bark or meow
 Persistently dilated pupils
 Facial muscle weakness
 Aspiration pneumonia

Myositis and Myopathies

DIFFERENTIAL DIAGNOSIS
 Inflammatory Myopathies
 Masticatory myositis
 • Immunoglobulin G (IgG) antibodies to type 2M
 myofibers

- German Shepherd, retrievers, and Doberman Pinscher predisposed
- Young to middle-aged dogs

Canine idiopathic polymyositis
- Large-breed dogs predisposed

Feline idiopathic polymyositis

Dermatomyositis
- Herding breeds, especially Shetland Sheepdog and Collie

Protozoal myositis
- *Toxoplasma gondii* infection
- *Neospora caninum* infection

Metabolic Myopathies

Glucocorticoid excess
- Hyperadrenocorticism
- Exogenous corticosteroids

Hypothyroidism

Hypokalemic polymyopathy (cat)
- Increased urinary excretion
- Decreased dietary intake

Inherited Myopathies

Muscular dystrophy
- Hereditary Labrador Retriever muscular dystrophy

Myotonia—Chow Chow, Staffordshire Bull Terrier, Labrador Retriever, Rhodesian Ridgeback, Great Dane, others

Malignant hyperthermia
- Hypermetabolic disorder of skeletal muscle
- Genetic defect in intracellular calcium homeostasis

Neurologic Examination

COMPONENTS

Mental State
Normal
Depression
Stupor
Coma
Agitation
Delirium

Posture
Normal, upright
Head tilt
Wide-based stance
Recumbent
Extensor posturing

Gait
Proprioceptive deficits
Paresis
Circling
Ataxia
Dysmetria
Lameness

Postural Reactions
Conscious proprioception
Hopping
Wheelbarrowing
Hemiwalking

Muscle Tone
Atrophy
Decreased muscle tone (lesions of lower motor neurons)
Increased muscle tone (lesions of upper motor neurons)
Schiff-Sherrington posture (increased muscle tone and
hyperextension of thoracic limbs)

Spinal Reflexes
Absent, depressed, normal, or exaggerated
Thoracic limb withdrawal (sixth cervical [C6], C7, C8,
first thoracic [T1])
Patellar (fourth lumbar [L4], L5, L6)
Pelvic limb withdrawal (L6, L7, first sacral [S1])
Sciatic (L6, L7, S1)
Cranial tibial (L6, L7)
Perineal (S1, S2, S3, pudendal nerve)
Bulbourethral (S1, S2, S3, pudendal nerve)
Panniculus (response absent caudal to spinal cord lesion,
used at T3-L3)

Sensation and Pain
Superficial pain
Deep pain
Hyperesthesia

Urinary Tract Function

Cranial Nerves

Peripheral Neuropathies

Clinical signs depend on the nerve affected and the severity of the lesion.

DIFFERENTIAL DIAGNOSIS
Focal Disease
Trauma
Mechanical blows
Fractures
Pressure
Stretching
Laceration
Injection of agents into nerves

Peripheral Nerve Tumors
Schwannoma
Neurofibroma
Neurofibrosarcoma
Lymphoma

Facial Nerve Paralysis
Otitis media
Trauma
Neoplasia
Foreign body (e.g., grass awn)
Nasopharyngeal polyp in cats
Hypothyroidism
Idiopathic

Trigeminal Nerve Paralysis
Bilateral, idiopathic disorder, often self-limiting

Idiopathic Peripheral Vestibular Disease

Hyperchylomicronemia
Leads to xanthomas in skin
May compress peripheral nerves

Ischemic Neuromyopathy
Caudal aortic thromboembolism

Generalized Chronic Polyneuropathies

Idiopathic

Metabolic disorders

- Diabetes mellitus
- Hypothyroidism

Paraneoplastic syndromes

- Insulinoma
- Other tumors

Systemic lupus erythematosus (SLE) or other immune-mediated disease

Chronic organophosphate toxicity

Generalized Acute Neuropathies

Acute polyradiculoneuritis ("coonhound paralysis")

Disorders of neuromuscular junction

- Botulism
- Tick paralysis
- Myasthenia gravis

Protozoal polyradiculoneuritis

Dysautonomia

Developmental/Congenital Neuropathies

Loss of motor neurons—Cairn Terrier, German Shepherd, English Pointer, Rottweiler, Swedish Lapland, Brittany Spaniel

Loss of peripheral axons—German Shepherd, Alaskan Malamute, Birman cat, Rottweiler, Boxer, Dalmatian

Schwann cell dysfunction—Golden Retriever, Tibetan Mastiff

Loss of sensory neuron of axon and laryngeal nerves—Dachshund, English Pointer, Shorthaired Pointer, Bouvier des Flandres, Siberian Husky

Inborn errors of metabolism

- Hyperchylomicronemia (cat)
- Hyperoxaluria type 2 (shorthaired cat)
- α-L-Fucosidosis (English Springer Spaniel)
- Atypical GM2 gangliosidosis (cat)
- Globoid cell leukodystrophy
- Niemann-Pick disease (Siamese)
- Glycogen storage disease (Norwegian forest cat)

Spinal Cord Disease

DIFFERENTIAL DIAGNOSIS

Acute
Trauma
Hemorrhage/coagulopathy
Infarction
Type I intervertebral disk herniation
Fibrocartilaginous embolism

Subacute/Progressive
Diskospondylitis
Noninfectious inflammatory diseases
- Corticosteroid-responsive meningitis/arteritis
- Granulomatous meningoencephalitis
- Feline polioencephalomyelitis

Infectious inflammatory diseases
- Bacterial, fungal, rickettsial, protothecal, protozoal, nematodiasis

Distemper myelitis
Feline infectious peritonitis (FIP) meningitis/myelitis

Chronic Progressive
Neoplasia
Type II intervertebral disk protrusion
Degenerative myelopathy
Cauda equina syndrome
    Cervical vertebral malformation/malarticulation
    (wobbler syndrome)
Lumbosacral vertebral canal stenosis
Spondylosis deformans
Hypervitaminosis A (cats)
Dural ossification
Diffuse idiopathic skeletal hyperostosis
Synovial cyst

Progressive in Young Animals
Neuronal abiotrophies and degenerations
Metabolic storage diseases
Atlantoaxial luxation
Congenital vertebral anomalies

Congenital (Constant)
Spinal bifida
Congenital agenesis of Manx cats
Spinal dysraphism

Hereditary ataxia
Pilonidal, epidermoid, and dermoid cysts
Syringomyelia/hydromyelia

Spinal Cord Lesions

LOCALIZATION
Cranial Cervical Lesion (C1-C5)
Upper motor neuron (UMN) signs in rear limbs
UMN signs in forelimbs

Caudal Cervical Lesion (C6-T2)
UMN signs in rear limbs
Lower motor neuron (LMN) signs in forelimbs

Thoracolumbar Lesion (T3-L3)
UMN signs in rear limbs
Normal forelimbs

Lumbosacral Lesion (L4-S3)
LMN signs in rear limbs
Loss of perineal sensation and reflexes
Normal forelimbs

Sacral Lesion (S1-S3)
Normal forelimbs
Normal patellar reflexes
Loss of sciatic function
Loss of perineal sensation and reflexes

Systemic Disease

NEUROLOGIC MANIFESTATIONS
Oxygen Deprivation
Vascular Disease
Ischemia
Thromboembolic disease
Shock
Cardiac disease

Hemorrhage
Vessel rupture secondary to hypertension
Coagulopathy
Vasculitis

Hypoxia
Pulmonary disease
Decreased oxygen transport
Heart failure

Hypoglycemia
Decreased Output or Metabolism
Primary liver disease
Malnutrition
Thiamine deficiency

Increased Uptake
Hyperinsulinemia
Islet cell tumors
Insulin overdose

Non–Islet Cell Neoplasia
Hepatoma
Leiomyoma

Excessive Metabolism
Sepsis
Breed or activity-related

Increased Uptake of Amino Acids by Extrahepatic Tissues

Water and Ionic Imbalances
Water
Hypoosmolar States (Retention of Free Water)
Hyponatremia

Hyperosmolar States (Loss of Free Water)
Hypernatremia (diabetes insipidus)
Hyperglycemia (diabetes mellitus)

Ions (Excess or Deficiency)
Calcium
Potassium

Endogenous Neurotoxins
Renal Toxins

Hepatoencephalopathy

Endocrine Disease
Adrenal
Hyperadrenocorticism
Hypoadrenocorticism

Adrenergic Dysregulation
Pheochromocytoma

Thyroid
Hypothyroidism
- Myxedema
- Neuromyopathy

Thyrotoxicosis
- Hyperthyroidism
- Iatrogenic

Exogenous Neurotoxins
Plant toxins

Sedative depressant drugs (e.g., antiepileptic drugs)

Heat stroke

Remote Neurologic Manifestations of Cancer
Metastasis to the nervous system

Vascular accidents and infection

Adverse effects of therapy

Paraneoplastic syndromes

Vestibular Disease

CLINICAL FINDINGS
Central and Vestibular Disease
Head tilt to side of lesion

Falling/rolling to side of lesion

Vomiting, salivation

Incoordination

Ventral strabismus on side of lesion (±)

Nystagmus, fast phase away from lesion

Nystagmus may intensify with changes in body position.

Peripheral Vestibular Disease
Nystagmus is horizontal or rotatory.

No change in nystagmus direction with changes in head position

Postural reactions and proprioception normal

Concurrent Horner's syndrome, cranial nerve VII paralysis with middle/inner ear involvement; other cranial nerves normal

Central Vestibular Disease

Nystagmus horizontal, rotatory, or vertical

Nystagmus direction may change direction with change in head position.

Abnormal postural reactions and proprioception may be seen on side of lesion.

Multiple cranial nerve deficits may be seen.

Ocular Disorders

Blindness, Acute

DIFFERENTIAL DIAGNOSIS, DOGS AND CATS

Cornea
Edema (glaucoma, trauma, endothelial dystrophy, immune-mediated keratitis, neurotropic keratitis)
Cellular infiltrate (bacterial, viral, fungal)
Vascular invasion (exposure keratitis)
Fibrosis (scar formation)
Dystrophy (lipid, genetic)

Aqueous humor
Fibrin (anterior uveitis: many etiologies)
Hyphema (trauma, coagulopathies, neoplasia)

Lens
Cataracts (genetic, diabetes, metabolic, toxic, traumatic, nutritional)

Vitreous
Hemorrhage (trauma, systemic hypertension, retinal detachment, neoplasia, coagulopathy)
Hyalitis (numerous infectious agents, penetrating injury)

Retina
Retinopathy (glaucoma, sudden acquired retinal degeneration [SARD], progressive retinal atrophy, central progressive retinal atrophy, feline central retinal atrophy, toxicity)
Retinal detachment (neoplasia, retinal dysplasia, hereditary/congenital, exudative/transudative disorders such as systemic hypertension or infection-induced inflammatory disease)

Lesions that Prevent Transmission of the Image

Viruses (canine distemper, feline infectious peritonitis [FIP])

Systemic diseases (neoplasia, traumatic avulsion of optic nerve, granulomatous meningoencephalitis, hydrocephalus, optic nerve hypoplasia, immune-mediated optic neuritis, systemic mycoses)

Lesions that Prevent Interpretation of the Visual Message

Canine distemper, FIP, granulomatous meningoencephalitis, systemic mycoses, trauma, heat stroke, hypoxia, hydrocephalus, hepatoencephalopathy, neoplasia, storage diseases, postictal, meningitis

Ocular Manifestations of Systemic Diseases

SURFACE OCULAR DISEASE

Eyelids

Immunosuppressive disorders may predispose to meibomian gland infection with *Demodex* or *Staphylococcus* spp.

Eyelids have mucocutaneous junction; affected by autoimmune disorders such as systemic lupus erythematosus (SLE) and pemphigoid diseases; also may be affected by uveodermatologic syndrome and vasculitis.

Altered lid position, cranial nerve III or VII dysfunction

Horner's syndrome: decreased sympathetic tone causing enophthalmos with third eyelid protrusion, ptosis, and miosis; often idiopathic; may be seen with disease of brain, spinal cord, brachial plexus, thorax, mediastinum, neck, temporal bone, tympanic bulla, or orbit.

Conjunctivitis

May reflect disease of deeper ocular structures

Good location to detect pallor, cyanosis, icterus

Feline herpesvirus type 1 (FHV-1) and *Chlamydophila felis* are primary pathogens of the conjunctiva.

Cornea/Sclera

Creamy pink discoloration of cornea may be seen with lymphoma.

Corneal lipidosis appears similar; may be secondary to hyperlipidemia from hypothyroidism, hyperadrenocorticism, diabetes mellitus, and familial hypertriglyceridemia.

Keratoconjunctivitis Sicca
Most cases are caused by lymphoplasmacytic dacryoadenitis.

Rarely seen with xerostomia (Sjögren's-like syndrome)

Possible causes include drug therapy, atropine, sulfa drugs, etodolac, and anesthetic agents.

Others causes include canine distemper, FHV-1, and dysautonomia.

UVEAL TRACT, LENS, FUNDUS
Uveal Tract
Hyphema or Hemorrhage
Hypertension, rickettsial disease, trauma, coagulopathy, lymphoma, metastatic neoplasia

Protein or Fibrin Deposition
Trauma, feline infectious peritonitis (FIP), uveodermatologic syndrome, lens capsule rupture, rickettsial disease

Cellular (Hypopyon) or Granulomatous Infiltrates
Trauma, lymphoma, metastatic neoplasia, uveodermatologic syndrome, algae or yeast, lens capsule rupture, FIP, systemic mycoses, toxoplasmosis

Other infectious agents associated with uveal tract disease include feline immunodeficiency virus (FIV), feline leukemia virus (FeLV), mycobacteria, FHV-1, *Bartonella* spp., *Ehrlichia* spp., *Leishmania donovani*, *Rickettsia rickettsii*, *Brucella canis*, *Leptospira* spp., and canine adenovirus.

Iris Abnormalities (Papillary Changes)
Anisocoria with FeLV

Miosis with Horner's syndrome

Mydriasis with dysautonomia

Lens
Cataracts
Most common cause in dogs is hereditary.

Cataracts are frequent complication of diabetes mellitus.

Uveitis may also cause cataracts (most common cause in cats).

Other causes include hypocalcemia (hypoparathyroidism), electric shock, lightning strike, altered nutrition (e.g., puppies fed milk replacer).

Lens Luxation/Subluxation

Most often secondary to severe intraocular disease (uveitis)

May be primary in terriers

Fundus

Usually affected by diseases that extend from the uveal tract (see previous section) or from central nervous system (immune-mediated diseases such as granulomatous meningoencephalitis or neoplasia of CNS).

Papilledema

Optic nerve edema without hemorrhage, exudates, or blindness

Seen with increased intracranial pressure

Taurine Deficiency

Retinal degeneration

May also cause dilated cardiomyopathy

Retinal Visualization

Allows assessment of systemic condition, including anemia (attenuated, pale vessels), hyperlipidemia (creamy orange hue to vessels), hyperviscosity (increased vessel tortuosity)

Systemic Hypertension

Causes extravasation of blood into retina, choroid, or subretinal space

Toxicology

Chemical Toxicoses
Plant Toxicoses
Venomous Bites and Stings

Chemical Toxicoses

TOXICANTS

Kerosene, Gasoline, Mineral Seal Oil, Turpentine, Others

Pulmonary, central nervous system (CNS), and gastrointestinal (GI) signs: may lead to hepatotoxicity, renal toxicity, and cardiac arrhythmias

Naphthalene (Mothballs)

Vomiting, lethargy, seizures, acute Heinz body hemolytic anemia, methemoglobinemia, hemoglobinuria, renal failure

Ethanol, Methanol (Wood Alcohol)

CNS depression, behavioral changes, ataxia, hypothermia, respiratory and cardiac arrest

Ethylene Glycol

Early intoxication: ataxia, progresses to oliguric renal failure with renomegaly, vomiting, hypothermia, coma, and death

Propylene Glycol

Ataxia, CNS depression

Phenol Products (Household Cleaners)

Cats particularly sensitive; hepatic and renal damage, ataxia, weakness, tremors, coma, seizures, respiratory alkalosis

Anticoagulant Rodenticides

Petechiae, ecchymosis, weakness, pallor, respiratory distress, CNS depression, hematemesis, epistaxis, melena, ataxia, paresis, seizures, sudden death

Zinc Phosphate

Anorexia, lethargy, weakness, abdominal pain, vomiting early after ingestion, progresses to recumbency, tremors, seizures, cardiopulmonary collapse, death

Cholecalciferol (Vitamin D) Rodenticides and Medications

Anorexia, CNS depression, vomiting, muscle weakness, constipation, bloody diarrhea, polyuria/polydipsia

Bromethalin Rodenticides

High-dose exposure: muscle tremors, hyperexcitability, vocalization, seizures, hyperesthesia, vomiting, dyspnea

Pyrethrin and Pyrethroid Insecticides

CNS depression, hypersalivation, muscle tremors, vomiting, ataxia, dyspnea, anorexia, hypothermia, hyperthermia, seizures, rarely death

Organophosphate and Carbamate Insecticides

Muscarinic signs (salivation, lacrimation, bronchial secretion, vomiting, diarrhea) and nicotinic signs (muscle tremors, respiratory paralysis), mixed signs (CNS depression, seizures, miosis, hyperactivity)

2,4-Dichlorophenoxyacetic Acid

Vomiting, diarrhea; greater exposure may cause CNS depression, ataxia, and hindlimb myotonia.

Lead (Paints, Batteries, Linoleum, Solder, Plumbing Supplies, fishing Weights)

High-level exposure: vomiting, abdominal pain, anorexia, diarrhea, megaesophagus
CNS signs, behavioral changes, hysteria, ataxia, tremors, opisthotonos, blindness, seizures

Zinc

Acute ingestion: vomiting, CNS depression, lethargy, diarrhea
Chronic exposure: anorexia, vomiting, diarrhea, CNS depression, pica, hemolysis, regenerative anemia, spherocytosis, inflammatory leukogram, icterus, renal failure

Iron

Vomiting, diarrhea, abdominal pain, hematemesis, melena; rarely, progresses to multisystemic failure

Plant Toxicoses

PLANTS THAT CAUSE HEMOLYSIS
 Onion

PLANTS THAT AFFECT THE CARDIOVASCULAR SYSTEM
 Cardiac glycoside toxicity: bradycardia with first-, second-,
  or third-degree atrioventricular (AV) block, ventricular
  arrhythmias, asystole, and sudden death; also see
  gastrointestinal (GI) signs
   Common oleander *(Nerium oleander)*
   Yellow oleander *(Thevetia peruviana)*
   Foxglove *(Digitalis purpurea)*
   Lily of the valley *(Convallaria majalis)*
   Kalanchoe *(Bryophyllum* spp.)
 Azalea *(Rhododendron* spp.): weakness, hypotension,
  dyspnea, respiratory failure, GI signs
 Yew *(Taxus* spp.): conduction disturbances, bradycardia, GI
  signs, weakness, seizures; poor prognosis once signs are
  seen

PLANTS AFFECTING THE GASTROINTESTINAL SYSTEM
 Oxalate-containing plants: gastric and ocular irritants
   Dumbcane *(Dieffenbachia* spp.)
   Philodendron *(Philodendron* spp.)
   Peace lily *(Spathiphyllum* spp.)
   Devil's ivy *(Epiprennum aureum)*
   Rhubarb leaves *(Rheum* spp.)
 Philodendron may cause renal and central nervous system
  (CNS) signs in cats.
 Chinaberry tree *(Melia azedarach)*: vomiting, diarrhea,
  abdominal pain, hypersalivation, may progress to CNS
  signs and death
 Cycad palms *(Cycas* spp.) or sago palms *(Macrozamia* spp.):
  vomiting, diarrhea, followed by lethargy, depression,
  liver failure, and death (dogs)
 English ivy *(Hedera helix)*: GI irritation, profuse salivation,
  abdominal pain, vomiting, diarrhea
 Castor bean plant *(Ricinus communis)*: ricin is among the
  most deadly poisons in the world; severe abdominal
  pain, vomiting, diarrhea, seizures, cerebral edema;
  prognosis for recovery is poor once clinical signs
  develop.
 Holly *(Ilex* spp.), poinsettia *(Euphorbia pulcherrima)*, mistletoe
  (Phoradendron flavescens): mild GI irritation, occasionally
  diarrhea, more serious effects with mistletoe

Amaryllis, jonquil, daffodil (family Amaryllidaceae), tulip (family Liliaceae), iris (family Iridaceae): ingestion of bulb associated with mild to moderate gastroenteritis

Autumn crocus *(Colchinum autumnale)*, glory lily *(Gloriosa* spp.): colchicine, vomiting, diarrhea, abdominal pain, hypersalivation progressing to depression, multiple organ system collapse and death

Solanaceae family: tomato, eggplant, deadly or black nightshade, Jerusalem cherry-solanine, gastric irritant; may cause CNS depression and cardiac arrhythmias; nightshade can also contain belladonna.

Mushrooms: amanitine poisoning *(Amanita virosa, Amanita phalloides, Conocybe filaris)*, orellanine poisoning *(Cortinarius orellanus, Cortinarius rainierensis)*, monomethylhydrazine *(Gyromitra esculenta)*—severe hepatic disease; survivors of hepatic phase may succumb to renal tubular necrosis.

PLANTS AFFECTING THE NEUROLOGIC SYSTEM

Tobacco *(Nicotiana tabacum)*: vomiting, CNS involvement, cardiac involvement

Hallucinogenic plants: psilocybins or "magic mushrooms," marijuana *(Cannabis sativa)*, jimsonweed *(Datura stramonium)*, thorn apple *(Datura metaliodyl)*, blue morning glory *(Ipomoea violacea)*, nutmeg *(Myristica fragrans)*, peyote (family Cactaceae)

Nettle toxicity (family Urticaceae): hunting dogs, toxins contained in needles (histamine, acetylcholine, serotonin, formic acid), salivation, vomiting, pawing at mouth, tremors, dyspnea, slow and irregular heartbeat

Macadamia nuts: locomotor disturbances, tremors, ataxia, weakness

PLANTS AFFECTING THE RENAL SYSTEM

Easter lily (*Lilium longiflorum*) and daylily (*Hemerocallis* spp.), possibly other lilies: toxic to cats, vomiting, depression, anorexia, leading to acute renal failure, poor prognosis without early treatment

Raisins/grapes: acute renal failure

PLANTS CAUSING SUDDEN DEATH

Seeds of many fruit trees (apple, apricot, cherry, peach, plum), contain cyanogenic glycosides

Venomous Bites and Stings

SNAKES, SPIDERS, OTHERS

Crotalids (Pit Vipers, Rattlesnakes, Copperhead, Water Moccasin)

Enzymatic and nonenzymatic proteins, local tissue damage: localized pain, salivation, weakness, fasciculations, hypotension, alterations in respiratory pattern, regional lymphadenopathy, mucosal bleeding, obtundation, convulsions, anemia, echinocytosis, stress leukogram

Elapids (Coral Snakes)

Rare envenomation, signs delayed 10-18 hours, emesis, salivation, agitation, central depression, quadriplegia, hyporeflexia, intravascular hemolysis, respiratory paralysis

Latrodectus spp. (Widow Spiders)

Hyperesthesia, muscle fasciculations, cramping, somatic abdominal pain (characteristic sign)

Loxoscelidae (Recluse or Brown Spiders)

Cutaneous form: bull's-eye lesion, pale center with localized thrombosis, surrounded by erythema, develops into a hemorrhagic bulla with underlying eschar

Viscerocutaneous form: Coombs-negative hemolytic anemia, thrombocytopenia, disseminated intravascular coagulation (DIC)

Tick Paralysis

Dermacentor and *Haemaphysalis* ticks, ascending paralysis, lower motor neuron signs, megaesophagus and aspiration pneumonia in severe cases, spontaneous recovery a few days after tick removal

Hymenopteran Stings

Bites and stings of winged insects and fire ants

Toxic and allergic reactions (localized angioedema, urticaria, emesis, diarrhea, hematochezia, respiratory depression, death)

Helodermatidae Lizard (Gila Monster)

Salivation, lacrimation, emesis, tachypnea, respiratory distress, tachycardia, hypotension, shock

Urogenital Disorders

Glomerular Disease

TYPES, DOGS AND CATS
  Glomerulonephritis
    Membranoproliferative form
    • Type I (mesangiocapillary)
    • Type II (dense deposit disease)
    Proliferative glomerulonephritis (mesangial and
      endocapillary)
    Crescentic type (rare)
  Amyloidosis
  Glomerulosclerosis
  Hereditary nephritis
  Immunoglobulin A (IgA) nephropathy
  Lupus nephritis
  Membranous glomerulopathy (most common in cats)
  Minimal change glomerulopathy

DIFFERENTIAL DIAGNOSIS FOR DISEASES ASSOCIATED WITH
GLOMERULAR DISEASE, DOGS
  Infection
    Bacterial
      Pyelonephritis
      Pyoderma
      Pyometra
      Endocarditis
      Bartonellosis

Brucellosis
Borreliosis
Other chronic bacterial infections

Parasitic
Dirofilariasis

Rickettsial
Ehrlichiosis

Fungal
Blastomycosis
Coccidioidomycosis

Protozoal
Babesiosis
Hepatozoonosis
Leishmaniasis
Trypanosomiasis

Viral
Canine adenovirus (type I) infection

Inflammation
Periodontal disease
Chronic dermatitis
Pancreatitis
Inflammatory bowel disease
Polyarthritis
Systemic lupus erythematosus (SLE)
Other immune-mediated diseases

Neoplasia
Lymphosarcoma
Mastocytosis
Leukemia
Systemic histiocytosis
Primary erythrocytosis
Other neoplasms

Miscellaneous
Corticosteroid excess
Trimethoprim-sulfa therapy
Hyperlipidemia
Chronic insulin infusion
Congential C3 deficiency
Cyclic hematopoiesis in gray collies

Familial
  Amyloidosis (Beagle, English Foxhound)
  Hereditary nephritis (Bull Terrier, English Cocker Spaniel,
    Dalmatian, Samoyed)
  Glomerulosclerosis (Doberman Pinscher, Newfoundland)
  Glomerular vasculopathy and necrosis (Greyhound)
  Mesangiocapillary glomerulonephritis (Bernese
    Mountain Dog)
  Atrophic glomerulopathy (Rottweiler)
  Proliferative and sclerosing glomerulonephritis (Soft-
    Coated Wheaten Terrier)

Idiopathic

DIFFERENTIAL DIAGNOSIS FOR DISEASES ASSOCIATED WITH GLOMERULAR DISEASE, CATS
Infection
  Bacterial
    Pyelonephritis
    Chronic bacterial infections
    Mycoplasmal polyarthritis

  Viral
    Feline immunodeficiency virus (FIV)
    Feline infectious peritonitis (FIP)
    Feline leukemia virus (FeLV)

Inflammation
  Pancreatitis
  Cholangiohepatitis
  Chronic progressive polyarthritis
  SLE
  Other immune-mediated diseases

Neoplasia
  Lymphosarcoma
  Leukemia
  Mastocytosis
  Other neoplasms

Miscellaneous
  Acromegaly
  Mercury toxicity

Familial

Idiopathic

Prostatic Disease

DIFFERENTIAL DIAGNOSIS
Benign prostatic hyperplasia
Acute prostatitis
Chronic prostatitis
Abscess
Cyst
Prostatic neoplasia

Pyelonephritis, Bacterial

CLINICAL FINDINGS, DOGS AND CATS
Fever
Renal pain
Anorexia
Lethargy
Cellular casts in urine sediment
Azotemia
Inability to concentrate urine
Polyuria/polydipsia
Ultrasonographic or excretory urographic abnormalities
• Renal pelvis dilatation
• Asymmetric filling of diverticula
• Dilated ureters
Bacteria in inflammatory lesions on histopathologic
examination
Positive culture of ureteral urine collected by cystoscopy
Positive culture of urine obtained after rinsing bladder with
sterile saline
Positive culture of urine obtained by ultrasound-guided
pyelocentesis

Renal Disease (see also Glomerular Disease)

FAMILIAL—DOGS AND CATS
Amyloidosis—Beagle, English Foxhound, Shar-Pei,
Abyssinian cat, Oriental shorthaired cat, Siamese cat
Fanconi's syndrome (tubular dysfunction)—Basenji
Tubular dysfunction (renal glucosuria)—Norwegian
Elkhound

Basement membrane disorder—Bull Terrier, Doberman Pinscher, English Cocker Spaniel, Samoyed

Membranoproliferative glomerulonephritis—Bernese Mountain Dog, Brittany Spaniel, Soft-Coated Wheaten Terrier

Glomerular disease—Rottweiler, Beagle

Periglomerular fibrosis—Norwegian Elkhound

Polycystic kidney disease—Cairn Terrier, West Highland White Terrier, Bull Terrier, Persian cat

DIFFERENTIAL DIAGNOSIS, RENAL TUBULAR DISEASE

Cystinuria

Inherited proximal tubular defect

Many breeds of dogs, including mixed breeds

Often leads to cystine calculi formation

Carnitinuria

Reported in dogs with cystinuria

May lead to carnitine deficiency and cardiomyopathy

Hyperuricosuria

Abnormal purine metabolism

- Dalmatian
- Dogs with primary hepatic disease

May lead to urate urolithiasis

Hyperxanthinuria (rare)

Seen in dogs receiving allopurinol to prevent urate uroliths

Congenital hyperxanthinuria seen in a family of Cavalier King Charles Spaniels

Renal Glucosuria

Primary renal glucouria (rare)

- Scottish Terrier, Basenji, Norwegian Elkhound, mixed breeds

Fanconi's Syndrome

Inherited proximal tubular defect

Basenji most common

May lead to renal failure

Renal Tubular Acidosis

Rare tubular disorders that lead to hyperchloremic metabolic acidosis

- Proximal renal tubular acidosis
- Distal renal tubular acidosis

Nephrogenic Diabetes Insipidus

Any renal disorder that suppresses the kidneys' response
  to antidiuretic hormone (ADH)

Congenital (rare)

Acquired

- Toxic (*Escherichia coli* endotoxin)
- Drugs (glucocorticoids, chemotherapeutics)
- Metabolic disease (hypokalemia, hypercalcemia)
- Tubular injury or loss (polycystic renal disease,
  bacterial pyelonephritis)
- Medullary washout

RENAL TOXINS IN DOGS AND CATS

Therapeutic Agents

Antibacterial Agents

Aminoglycosides
Sulfonamides
Nafcillin
Penicillins
Cephalosporins
Fluoroquinolones
Carbapenems
Rifampin
Tetracyclines
Vancomycin

Antifungal Agents

Amphotericin B

Antiviral Agents

Acyclovir
Foscarnet

Antiprotozoal Agents

Pentamidine
Sulfadiazine
Trimethoprim-sulfamethoxazole
Dapsone

Anthelmintics

Thiacetarsamide

Cancer Chemotherapeutics

Cisplatin/carboplatin
Methotrexate
Doxorubicin
Azathioprine

Immunosuppressive Drugs
    Cyclosporine
    Interleukin-2

Nonsteroidal Antiinflammatory Drugs (NSAIDs)

Angiotensin-Converting Enzyme (ACE) Inhibitors

Diuretics

Miscellaneous Agents
    Dextran 40
    Allopurinol
    Cimetidine
    Apomorphine
    Deferoxamine
    Streptokinase
    Methoxyflurane
    Penicillamine
    Acetaminophen
    Tricyclic antidepressants

Radiocontrast Agents

Nontherapeutic Agents
    Heavy Metals
        Lead
        Mercury
        Cadmium
        Chromium

    Organic Compounds
        Ethylene glycol
        Carbon tetrachloride
        Chloroform
        Pesticides
        Herbicides
        Solvents

    Miscellaneous Agents
        Mushrooms
        Snake venom
        Grapes/raisins
        Bee venom
        Lily

Pigments
Hemoglobin/myoglobin

Hypercalcemia

CAUSES OF ACUTE RENAL FAILURE IN DOGS AND CATS
Primary Renal Disease
Infection
Pyelonephritis
Leptospirosis
Infectious canine hepatitis

Immune-Mediated Disease
Acute glomerulonephritis
Systemic lupus erythematosus (SLE)
Renal transplant rejection

Renal Neoplasia
Lymphoma

Nephrotoxicity
Exogenous toxins
Endogenous toxins
Drugs

Renal Ischemia
Prerenal Azotemia
Dehydration/hypovolemia
Deep anesthesia
Sepsis
Shock/vasodilation
Decreased oncotic pressure
Hyperthermia
Hypothermia
Hemorrhage
Burns
Transfusion reaction

Renal Vascular Disease
Avulsion
Thrombosis
Stenosis

Systemic Diseases with Renal Manifestations
Infection
• Bacterial endocarditis
• Feline infectious peritonitis (FIP)
• Borreliosis

- Babesiosis
- Leishmaniasis

Pancreatitis

Systemic inflammatory response syndrome (SIRS)

Sepsis

Multiple organ failure

Disseminated intravascular coagulation (DIC)

Heart failure

SLE

Hepatorenal syndrome

Malignant hypertension

Hyperviscosity syndrome

- Polycythemia
- Multiple myeloma

Urinary outflow obstruction

CAUSES OF CHRONIC RENAL FAILURE IN DOGS AND CATS

Inflammatory/infectious

- Pyelonephritis
- Leptospirosis
- Blastomycosis
- Leishmaniasis
- FIP

Familial/congenital (see p. 221)

Amyloidosis

Neoplasia

- Lymphosarcoma
- Renal cell carcinoma
- Nephroblastoma
- Others

Nephrotoxicants (see p. 225)

Renal ischemia

Sequela of acute renal failure

Glomerulopathies (see p. 218)

Nephrolithiasis

Bilateral hydronephrosis

- Spay granulomas
- Transitional cell carcinoma at trigone obstructing both ureters
- Nephrolithiasis

Polycystic kidney disease

Urinary outflow obstruction

Idiopathic

Reproductive Disorders

INFERTILITY—DIFFERENTIAL DIAGNOSIS, CANINE FEMALE
Normal Cycles
Improper breeding management
Infertile male
Elevated diestrual progesterone
- Early embryonic death
- Lesions in tubular system (vagina, uterus, uterine tubes)
- Placental lesions (brucellosis, herpes)

Normal diestrual progesterone
- Cystic follicles (ovulation failure)

Abnormal Cycles
Abnormal Estrus
Will Not Copulate
Not in estrus
Inexperience
Partner preference
Vaginal anomaly
Hypothyroidism (possibly)

Prolonged Estrus
Cystic follicles
Ovarian neoplasia
Exogenous estrogens

Short Estrus
Observation error
Geriatric

Abnormal Interestrual Interval
Prolonged Interval
Photoperiod (queen)
Pseudopregnant/pregnant (queen)
Normal breed variation
Glucocorticoids (bitch)
Old age
Luteal cysts

Short Interval
Normal (especially queen)
Ovulation failure (especially queen)
Corpus luteum failure

"Split heat" (bitch)
Exogenous drugs

Not Cycling
Prepubertal
Ovariohysterectomy
Estrus suppressants
Silent heat
Unobserved heat
Photoperiod (queen)
Intersex (bitch)
Ovarian dysgenesis
Hypothyroidism (possibly)
Glucocorticoid excess
Hypothalamic-pituitary disorder
Geriatric

INFERTILITY—DIFFERENTIAL DIAGNOSIS, CANINE MALE

Inflammatory Ejaculate
Prostatitis
Orchitis
Epididymitis

Azoospermia
Sperm-rich fraction not collected
Sperm not ejaculated
- Incomplete ejaculation
- Obstruction
- Prostate swelling
Sperm not produced
- Endocrine
- Testicular
- Metabolic disorders

Abnormal Motility/Abnormal Morphology
Iatrogenic
Prepubertal
Poor ejaculation
Long abstinence

Abnormal Libido
Female not in estrus
Behavioral
Pain
Geriatric

Normal Libido
Improper stud management
Infertile female

Normal Libido/Abnormal Mating Ability
Orthopedic
Neurologic
Prostatic disease
Penile problem
Prepuce problem

PENIS, PREPUCE, AND TESTES DISORDERS—DIFFERENTIAL DIAGNOSIS

Acquired Penile Disorders
Penile trauma
- Hematoma
- Laceration
- Fracture of os penis

Priapism (abnormal, persistent erection)
Neoplasia
Vesicles
Warts
Ulcers

Congenital Penile Disorders
Persistent penile frenulum
Penile hypoplasia
Hypospadias (defect in closure of urethra)
Diphallia (duplication of penis)

Preputial Disorders
Balanoposthitis
- Bacteria infection
- Blastomycosis
- Canine herpesvirus

Phimosis
Paraphimosis

Testicular Disorders
Cryptorchidism
Orchitis/epididymitis
- *Mycoplasma* spp.
- *Brucella canis*
- *Blastomyces* spp.
- *Ehrlichia* spp.
- Rocky Mountain spotted fever
- Feline infectious peritonitis (FIP)

Testicular torsion
Testicular neoplasia
- Sertoli cell tumor
- Leydig cell tumor
- Seminoma

DRUGS AND METABOLIC DISORDERS AFFECTING MALE REPRODUCTION

Glucocorticoids (hyperadrenocorticism, exogenous glucocorticoids)
> Decreased luteinizing hormone (LH), testosterone, sperm output, seminal volume, and libido; increased sperm abnormalities

Estrogens, androgens, anabolic steroids
> Decreased LH, testosterone, and spermatogenesis

Cimetidine
> Decreased testosterone, libido, and sperm count

Spironolactone, anticholinergics, propranolol, digoxin, verapamil, thiazide diuretics, chlorpromazine, barbiturates, diazepam, phenytoin, primidone
> Decreased testosterone and libido

Progestagens, ketoconazole
> Decreased testosterone

Amphoterin B, many anticancer drugs
> Decreased spermatogenesis

Diabetes mellitus
> Decreased libido and sperm count, abnormal semen

Renal failure, stress
> Decreased libido and sperm count

Ureteral Diseases

DIFFERENTIAL DIAGNOSIS

Vesicoureteral Reflux

Primary: 7-12 weeks old—intrinsic maldevelopment of ureterovesical junction, self-limiting
Secondary to lower urinary tract obstruction, urinary tract infection, surgical damage, neurologic disease of bladder, ectopic ureters

Congenital Anomalies

Ectopic ureters
Ureterocele

Ureter agenesis
Ureter duplication

Acquired Ureteral Disease
Ureteral trauma
- Blunt trauma
- Penetrating trauma
- Iatrogenic damage during surgery

Inadvertent ligation and transection during
   ovariohysterectomy
Urinoma (paraureteral pseudocyst)
Ureteral obstruction
- Intraluminal (blood clot, calculus)
- Intramural (fibrosis, stricture, neoplasia)
- Extramural (retroperitoneal mass, bladder neoplasia,
  inadvertent ligature)

Calculi
- Calcium oxalate (most common in cat)
- Struvite (both struvite and calcium oxalate are most
  common in dog)

Neoplasia
- Transitional cell carcinoma
- Leiomyoma
- Leiomyosarcoma
- Benign papilloma

Urinary Tract Infection (UTI)

CLINICAL FINDINGS
Lower UTI
Dysuria
Pollakiuria
Urge incontinence
Gross hematuria at end of micturition
Cloudy urine
Foul odor to urine
Small, painful, thickened bladder
Palpable urocystoliths
Pyuria
Hematuria
Proteinuria
Bacteruria

Upper UTI
Polyuria/polydipsia
Signs of systemic illness or infection
Possible renal failure
Fever
Abdominal pain
Kidneys normal to enlarged
Leukocytosis
Pyuria
Hematuria
Proteinuria
Bacteruria
Cellular or granular casts
Decreased urine specific gravity

Acute Prostatitis or Prostatic Abscess
Urethral discharge
Signs of systemic illness/infection
Fever
Painful prostate or abdomen
Prostatomegaly/asymmetry
Leukocytosis
Pyuria
Hematuria
Proteinuria
Bacteruria
Inflammatory prostatic cytology

Chronic Prostatitis
Recurrent UTIs
Urethral discharge
Possible dysuria
Normal complete blood count (CBC)
Pyuria
Hematuria
Proteinuria
Bacteruria
Prostatomegaly/asymmetry

CANINE LOWER URINARY TRACT DISEASE—DIFFERENTIAL DIAGNOSIS
Urocystoliths
Struvite (magnesium ammonium phosphate)
Calcium oxalate
Purine (urate/xanthine)
Cystine

Calcium phosphate
Silica
Compound uroliths

Urethral Obstruction

Urethroliths (see Urocystoliths)
Blood clots
Urethral stricture
Neoplasia
- Transitional cell carcinoma
- Prostatic adenocarcinoma
- Leiomyoma
- Leiomyosarcoma
- Prostatic adenocarcinoma
- Squamous cell carcinoma
- Myxosarcoma
- Lymphoma

Proliferative urethritis
Urinary bladder entrapment in perineal hernia
Trauma
- Penile fracture

Urinary Tract Trauma

Contusion (bladder or urethra)
Urethral tears
Rupture of bladder (blunt trauma, secondary to pelvic fracture, penetrating wound)
Avulsion of bladder or urethra
Penile fracture

Inflammation (Bladder or Urethra)

Bacterial UTI
Fungal UTI
Polypoid cystitis
Emphysematous cystitis
Cyclophosphamide-induced cystitis
Parasitic cystitis *(Capillaria plica)*

FELINE LOWER URINARY TRACT DISEASE—DIFFERENTIAL DIAGNOSIS

Feline idiopathic cystitis
Urethral plug
Urolithiasis
- Struvite
- Calcium oxalate
- Urate
- Cystine

Bacterial cystitis (less common in cats than in dogs)
Stricture
Neoplasia

Uroliths, Canine

CHARACTERISTICS

Calcium Oxalate Monohydrate or Dihydrate

Radiopaque
Acidic to neutral pH
Sharp projections or smooth uroliths; calcium oxalate
   dihydrate uroliths may be jackstone shaped.
Not associated with urinary tract infection
Calcium oxalate dihydrate crystals: square envelope
   shape
Calcium oxalate monohydrate crystals: dumbbell shaped

Struvite (Magnesium-Ammonium-Phosphate)

Radiopaque
Alkaline pH
Smooth to speculated if single; smooth and pyramidal in
   shape if multiple
Associated with infection with urease-producing bacteria
   (*Staphylococcus, Proteus, Mycoplasma* spp.)
"Coffin lid"–shaped crystals

Urate/Xanthine

Radiolucent to faintly radiopaque
Acidic pH
Smooth uroliths
Not associated with infection
Yellow-brown "thorn apple" (spherical) or amorphous
   crystals

Cystine

Faintly to moderately radiopaque
Acidic pH
Smooth, round uroliths; staghorn-shaped uroliths if
   nephroliths present
Not associated with infection
Hexagonal-shaped crystals

Calcium Phosphate
Radiopaque
Alkaline to normal pH for hydroxyapatite, acidic for
brushite
Small, variably shaped uroliths for hydroxyapatite
Smooth, round or pyramidal for brushite
Not associated with infection
Amorphous phosphate crystals or thin prisms (calcium
phosphate)

Silica
Radiopaque
Acidic to neutral pH
Jackstone-shaped uroliths
Not associated with infection
No crystals

Vaginal Discharge

DIFFERENTIAL DIAGNOSIS
Cornified Epithelial Cells
Normal proestrus
Normal estrus
Contamination of skin or epithelium
Abnormal source of estrogen
- Exogenous
- Ovarian follicular cyst
- Ovarian neoplasia

Mucus
Normal late diestrus of late pregnancy
Normal lochia
Mucometra
Androgenic stimulation

Neutrophils
Nonseptic (no microorganisms seen)
Vaginitis
Normal first day of diestrus
Metritis or pyometra

Septic
Vaginitis
Metritis

Pyometra
Abortion

Peripheral Blood
Subinvolution of placental sites
Uterine or vaginal neoplasia
Trauma to reproductive tract
Uterine torsion
Coagulopathies

Cellular Debris
Normal lochia
Abortion

PART THREE

Laboratory Values and Interpretation of Results

Note: Normal ranges are meant to provide the reader an approximation of normal. Individual laboratory values should be compared with the reference range values of the laboratory that performed the test.

Acetylcholine Receptor Antibody

Normal range:
Feline: < 0.3 nmol/L
Canine: < 0.6 nmol/L

Elevated in: myasthenia gravis

Note: A positive titer is diagnostic for myasthenia gravis. Negative titers occur in 10% to 20% of positive cases; therefore, a negative titer does not exclude myasthenia gravis.

Activated Coagulation Time (ACT)

Normal range:
Feline: 50-75 seconds
Canine: 60-110 seconds
   Screening test for intrinsic and common coagulation pathways (factors II, V, VIII, IX, X, XI, XII); may also be prolonged with severe thrombocytopenia and decreased fibrinogen.

Activated Partial Thromboplastin Time (APTT)

Normal range:
Feline: 10-25 seconds
Canine: 10-25 seconds
Determines abnormalities in the intrinsic coagulation pathway
Prolonged with deficiencies in factors VIII, IX, XI, XII and
   fibrinogen; also prolonged with disseminated intravascular
   coagulation (DIC)
Severely prolonged with hemophilia A (factor VIII deficiency)
   and hemophilia B (factor IX)

Adrenocorticotropic Hormone (ACTH), Endogenous

Normal range:
Feline: not reported
Canine: 10-70 pg/mL

Elevated in: pituitary-dependent hyperadrenocorticism

Decreased in: iatrogenic Cushing's syndrome and adrenal tumors

Adrenocorticotropic Hormone (ACTH) Stimulation Test

Normal range:
Pre-ACTH injection:
Feline: 1.0-4.5 µg/dL
Canine: 1.0-4.5 µg/dL

Post-ACTH injection:
Feline: 4.5-15.0 µg/dL
Canine: 5.5-20.0 µg/dL

Post-ACTH cortisol greater than 20.0 µg/dL in dogs and greater than 15 µg/dL in cats is suggestive of hyperadrenocorticism (Cushing's syndrome).

From 15% to 20% are false-negative results; false-positive results may be seen with stress or nonadrenal illness.

Pre-ACTH cortisol is in normal range and post-ACTH cortisol shows little to no change with iatrogenic Cushing's syndrome.

Pre-ACTH cortisol is below normal and post ACTH cortisol shows little change with hypoadrenocorticism.

Pre-ACTH and post-ACTH cortisol levels should be between 1 and 5 µg/dL with successful Lysodren induction or while on maintenance Lysodren therapy.

Note: ACTH stimulation does not differentiate pituitary-dependent hyperadrenocorticism from adrenal tumors. The low-dose dexamethasone test is more diagnostic for canine Cushing's syndrome.

Alanine Aminotransferase (ALT, Formerly SGPT)

Normal range:
Feline: 10-100 IU/L
Canine: 12-118 IU/L

Elevated in: hepatocellular membrane damage and leakage
Inflammation: chronic active hepatitis, lymphocytic/plasmacytic hepatitis (cats), enteritis, pancreatitis, peritonitis
Infection: bacterial hepatitis, leptospirosis, feline infectious peritonitis (FIP), infectious canine hepatitis
Toxicity: chemical, heavy metals, mycotoxins
Neoplasia: primary, metastatic
Drugs
Endocrine: diabetes mellitus, hyperadrenocorticism, hyperthyroidism
Trauma
Hypoxia: cardiopulmonary disease, thromboembolic disease
Metabolism: feline hepatic lipidosis, storage diseases
Liver lobe torsion
Hepatocellular regeneration

Decreased in: end-stage liver disease

Albumin

Normal range:
Feline: 2.5-3.9 g/dL
Canine: 2.7-4.4 g/dL

Elevated in: dehydration (globulin and total protein should also be increased), spurious (e.g., hemolysis, lipemia, lab error), higher in adult than in juveniles

Decreased in: protein-losing nephropathy (amyloidosis, glomerulonephritis, glomerulosclerosis), gastroenteropathy (malabsorption, maldigestion, protein-losing enteropathy), liver failure, malnutrition (dietary, parasitism), exudative skin disease (vasculitis, burns, abrasions, degloving injury), neonates, external blood loss, compensatory (chronic effusions, hyperglobulinemia, multiple myeloma)

Alkaline Phosphatase, Serum (SAP or ALP)

Normal range:
Feline: 6-102 IU/L
Canine: 5-131 IU/L

Elevated in: biliary tract abnormalities (pancreatitis, bile duct neoplasia, cholelithiasis, cholecystitis, ruptured gallbladder), hepatic parenchymal disease (cholangitis/cholangiohepatitis, chronic hepatitis, nodular hypoplasia, copper storage disease, hepatic lipidosis [cats], cirrhosis, hepatic neoplasia, [lymphoma, hemangiosarcoma, hepatocellular carcinoma, metastatic carcinoma], toxic hepatitis, feline infectious peritonitis [cats]), corticosteroids, anticonvulsants (phenobarbital, primidone), endocrine disorders (diabetes mellitus, hyperadrenocorticism [dogs], hyperthyroidism [cats]), enteritis, bone isoenzyme, young dog with bone growth, osteosarcoma, iatrogenic

Note: Almost any disorder that affects the liver can cause elevations in SAP levels.

Ammonia

Normal range:
Feline: 30-100 µg/dL
Canine: 45-120 µg/dL

Elevated in: hepatic failure (portosystemic shunt, cirrhosis), spurious (e.g., hemolysis, lipemia, lab error)

Note: Due to instability of samples, this test has been mostly been replaced by serum bile acids.

Amylase, Serum

Normal range:
Feline: 100-1200 U/L
Canine: 290-1125 U/L

Elevated in: pancreatitis, pancreatic neoplasia, pancreatic duct obstruction, pancreatic necrosis, enteritis, renal disease (decreased filtration of amylase)

Note: Serum amylase levels may not correlate with severity of disease.

Anion Gap

Normal range:
Feline: 12-24
Canine: 16.3-28.6

Laboratory calculation:
[Na + K] − [Cl + HCO$_3^-$] = Anion gap

Elevated in: toxicity (ethylene glycol, salicylates, other drugs [e.g., penicillins], alcohol), lactic acidosis (dehydration, shock, anoxia, cardiac arrest), metabolic acidosis, diabetic ketoacidosis, renal failure/uremia, hyperchloremic metabolic acidosis (renal tubular acidosis, severe diarrhea [loss of gastrointestinal bicarbonate]), hyperglobulinemia (multiple myeloma), gastrointestinal bicarbonate loss, severe hypercalcemia

Decreased in: hypoalbuminemia

Antinuclear Antibody (ANA)

Normal range:
Reported as a titer, very laboratory dependent. Refer to your lab for normal ranges.

High positive titer, with associated clinical and clinicopathologic signs, supports a diagnosis of systemic lupus erythematosus (SLE). Many inflammatory and infectious diseases and neoplasms can result in low positive titers. Results may be false negative with chronic glucocorticoid use.

Arterial Blood Gases

Normal range:

	CANINE	FELINE
pH	7.35-7.45	7.36-7.44
$PaCO_2$	36-44	28-32
PaO_2	90-100	90-100
TCO_2	25-27	21-23
HCO_3^-	24-26	20-22

Blood gas interpretation:

Evaluate PaO_2

Hypoxemia: arterial oxygen tension/partial pressure (PaO_2) of less than 85 mm Hg

Emergency treatment for hypoxemia needed when PaO_2 is less than 60 mm Hg.

Cyanosis may be seen when PaO_2 is 50 mm Hg or lower, depending on hemoglobin concentration.

Potential causes of hypoxemia

Right-left shunts (patent ductus arteriosus, ventricular septal defects, intrapulmonary shunts)

Ventilation/perfusion mismatch (various pulmonary diseases)

Diffusion impairment

Hypoventilation (anesthesia, neuromuscular disease, airway obstruction, central nervous system disease, pleural space or chest wall abnormality)

Decrease in fraction of inspired oxygen (hooked up to empty oxygen tank)

Evaluate pH

Increase in pH: alkalemia (metabolic alkalosis or respiratory alkalosis)

Decrease in pH: acidemia (metabolic acidosis or respiratory acidosis)

Assess acid-base status

If acidemic:

Arterial carbon dioxide tension ($PaCO_2$) elevated: respiratory acidosis

$PaCO_2$ decreased: compensatory respiratory alkalosis

Bicarbonate (HCO_3^-) decreased: metabolic acidosis

HCO_3^- elevated: compensatory metabolic alkalosis

If alkalotic:
Paco$_2$ decreased: respiratory alkalosis
Paco$_2$ elevated: compensatory respiratory acidosis
HCO$_3^-$ elevated: metabolic alkalosis
HCO$_3^-$ decreased: compensatory metabolic acidosis

Aspartate Aminotransferase (AST, Formerly SGOT)

Not considered clinically significant in the dog or cat.
Very sensitive but not very specific; significant amounts of AST found also in muscle.

Basophil Count

Normal range:
Feline: 0-150 cells/µL
Canine: 0-150 cells/µL

Elevated (basophilia) in: disorders associated with IgE production/binding (heartworm disease, atopy), inflammatory disease (gastrointestinal tract disease, respiratory tract disease), neoplasia (mast cell neoplasia, basophilic leukemia, lymphomatoid granulomatosis), associated with hyperlipoproteinemia and possibly hypothyroidism

Bicarbonate (HCO$_3^-$)

Normal range:
Feline: 20-22 mmol/L
Canine: 24-26 mmol/L

If acidemic:

Elevated in: metabolic alkalosis (with compensatory acidosis)

Decreased in: metabolic acidosis

If alkalotic:

Elevated in: metabolic alkalosis

Decreased in: metabolic acidosis (with compensatory alkalosis)

Bile Acids

Normal range:
Preprandial:
Feline and canine: 0-5.0 µmol/L

Postprandial:
Feline: 1-20.0 µmol/L
Canine: 5.0-25.0 µmol/L

Elevated in: hepatocellular disease, cholestatic disease, portosystemic shunt

Decreased in: delayed gastric emptying, malabsorption disorders, rapid intestinal transport

Patient must be fasted and cannot be icteric. Typically measure preprandial and 2-hour postprandial serum samples.

May also measure urine bile acids, although patients with portosystemic shunts tend to have lower urine bile acids than patients with hepatocellular disease.

Bilirubin

Normal range:
Feline: 0.1-0.4 mg/dL
Canine: 0.1-0.3 mg/dL

Elevated in: prehepatic, hemolytic anemia, cholestasis (extrahepatic [pancreatitis, cholangitis, cholecystitis, cholelithiasis, biliary neoplasia], intrahepatic [nodular hyperplasia, feline hepatic lipidosis, cholangitis/cholangiohepatitis, cirrhosis]), duodenal perforation, ruptured gallbladder

Blood Urea Nitrogen (BUN)

Normal range:
Feline: 14-36 mg/dL
Canine: 6-25 mg/dL

Elevated in: prerenal azotemia (dehydration, heart failure, shock, gastrointestinal hemorrhage, high-protein diet), increased catabolism (fever, drugs, [e.g., tetracycline]), renal failure, postrenal azotemia (urethral [obstruction, urolith, urethral tear, plant awn], bladder [obstruction, urolith, blood clot, polyp, neoplasia, rupture])

Decreased in: diuresis (polydipsia, hyperadrenocorticism, overzealous fluid therapy, drugs [e.g., glucocorticoids], diabetes insipidus), liver failure (portosystemic shunt, cirrhosis, urea cycle enzyme deficiency), low-protein diet, malnutrition, neonates

Buccal Mucosal Bleeding Time (BMBT)

Normal range:
Feline and canine: < 3 minutes
Prolonged bleeding time is a sensitive and specific indicator of diminished platelet function (e.g., von Willebrand's disease and uremia).

Calcium (Ca)

Normal range:
Feline: 8.2-10.8 mg/dL
Canine: 8.9-11.4 mg/dL

Elevated in: primary hyperparathyroidism, renal failure, hypoadrenocorticism, hypercalcemia of malignancy (lymphosarcoma, apocrine gland adenocarcinoma, carcinomas [nasal, mammary gland, gastric, thyroid, pancreatic, pulmonary], osteolytic [multiple myeloma, lymphosarcoma, squamous cell carcinoma, osteosarcoma, fibrosarcoma]), hypervitaminosis D (cholecalciferol rodenticides, plants, excessive supplementation), dehydration, granulomatous disease (systemic mycosis [blastomycosis], schistosomiasis, feline infectious peritonitis [FIP]), nonmalignant skeletal disorder (osteomyelitis, hypertrophic osteodystrophy [HOD]), iatrogenic disorder (excessive calcium supplementation, excessive oral phosphate binders), factitious disorders (serum lipemia, postprandial measurement, young animal), laboratory error, idiopathic (cats)

Decreased in: renal failure (acute and chronic), acute pancreatitis, intestinal malabsorption, primary hypoparathyroidism (idiopathic, post-thyroidectomy), puerperal tetany (eclampsia), ethylene glycol toxicity, hypoproteinemia/hypoalbuminemia, hypomagnesemia, nutritional secondary hyperparathyroidism, tumor lysis syndrome, phosphate-containing enemas, anticonvulsant medications, sodium bicarbonate administration, laboratory error

Cerebrospinal Fluid (CSF)

Normal range:

VALUE	CANINE	FELINE	CYTOLOGY (%)		
WBCs (× 10^3/L)	≤3	≤2	Monocytes	87	69-100
RBCs (× 10^6/L)	≤30	≤30	Lymphocytes	4	0-27
Protein (mg/dL)	≤33	≤36	Neutrophils	3	0-9
			Eosinophils	0	0
			Macrophages	6	0-3

Infectious central nervous system (CNS) disease: increased white blood cells (WBCs) and protein content

Inflammatory CNS disease: increased WBCs and protein content

Brain neoplasia: normal to mild elevation of WBCs, mild elevation of protein content

Hydrocephalus, lissencephaly: normal WBCs and protein content

Degenerative myelopathy, intervertebral disk disease, polyradiculoneuritis: normal WBCs and normal to mildly increased protein content

Chloride (Cl)

Normal range:
Feline: 104-128 mEq/L
Canine: 102-120 mEq/L

Elevated in: dehydration, metabolic acidosis, bromide therapy, intravenous saline administration

Decreased in: gastric vomiting, metabolic alkalosis, hypoadrenocorticism, diuretics (secondary to drug-induced polyuria), burns, syndrome of inappropriate secretion of antidiuretic hormone (ADH)

Cholesterol (CH)

Normal range:
Feline: 75-220 mg/dL
Canine: 92-324 mg/dL

Elevated in: postprandial, primary hyperlipidemia, endocrine disorders (hypothyroidism, hyperadrenocorticism, diabetes mellitus), cholestasis, dietary (high cholesterol diet), nephrotic syndrome, idiopathic (Doberman Pinscher, Rottweiler)

Decreased in: liver failure, malabsorption, maldigestion, protein-losing enteropathy, portosystemic shunt, lymphangiectasia, starvation, hypoadrenocorticism

Cholinesterase

Normal range:
Feline: 500-4000 U/L
Canine: 800-4000 U/L

Decreased in: organophosphate toxicity, carbamate toxicity

Cobalamin

Normal range:
Feline: 200-1680 pg/mL
Canine: 175-500 pg/mL

Decreased in: exocrine pancreatic insufficiency, distal small intestinal disease, diffuse small intestinal disease, small intestinal bacterial overgrowth (usually combined with an increased serum folate level)

Complete Blood Count (CBC)

Normal range:
Total white blood cell (WBC) count:

Feline: 3.5-16.0 $10^3/\mu L$
Canine: 4.0-15.5 $10^3/\mu L$

Total red blood cell (RBC) count:
Feline: 5.92-9.93 $10^6/\mu L$
Canine: 4.8-9.3 $10^6/\mu L$

Hemoglobin:
Feline: 9.3-15.9 g/dL
Canine: 12.1-20.3 g/dL

Hematocrit (packed cell volume):
Feline: 29%-48%
Canine: 36%-60%

Reticulocyte count:
Feline: 0-10.5% punctate or 0-1.0% aggregate
Canine: 0-1.0% aggregate

Mean corpuscular volume (MCV):
Feline: 37-61 fL
Canine: 58-79 fL

Mean corpuscular hemoglobin (MCH):
Feline: 11-21 pg
Canine: 19-28 pg

Mean corpuscular hemoglobin concentration (MCHC):
Feline: 30-38 g/dL
Canine: 30-38 g/dL

Platelet count:
Feline: 200-500 $10^3/\mu L$
Canine: 170-400 $10^3/\mu L$

Total solids:
Feline: 5.2-8.8 g/dL
Canine: 5.0-7.4 g/dL

Coombs' Test

Indicates presence of antibody and/or complement on the surface of erythrocytes; supports the diagnosis of immune-mediated hemolytic anemia.

Cortisol

Normal range:
Feline and canine: 1.0-4.5 µg/dL
    Not a reliable indicator of disease; considerable overlap between normal patients and those with adrenal disease.

Elevated in: stress (environmental, illness), drugs (prednisone and prednisolone [may cross-react in assay], anticonvulsants), pituitary- and adrenal-dependent hyperadrenocorticism

Decreased in: drugs (suppression of adrenal function), hypoadrenocorticism

Creatine Kinase (CK, formerly CPK)

Normal range:
Feline: 56-529 U/L
Canine: 59-895 U/L

Elevated in: trauma, myositis (immune mediated, eosinophilic myositis, masticatory muscle myositis, infectious [toxoplasmosis, neosporosis], endocarditis), exertional myositis, surgery (tissue damage), nutritional (hypokalemia [polymyopathy], taurine deficiency), prolonged recumbency, intramuscular injections, pyrexia, hypothermia, postinfarct ischemia (cardiomyopathy, disseminated intravascular coagulation [DIC])

Creatinine

Normal range:
Feline: 0.6-2.4 mg/dL
Canine: 0.5-1.6 mg/dL

Elevated in: azotemia (prerenal, renal, postrenal, rhabdomyolysis)

Decreased in: any condition that causes decreased muscle mass

Dexamethasone Suppression Tests

LOW-DOSE DEXAMETHASONE SUPPRESSION TEST (LDDST)

Normal: 4-hour cortisol level suppresses to less than 50% of baseline cortisol (usually less than 1.4 µg/dL), then 8-hour cortisol remains at or near that level.

Pituitary-dependent hyperadrenocorticism (PDH):
4-hour cortisol level is suppressed to less than 50% of baseline (60% of dogs) or less than 1.4 µg/dL (25% of dogs), and an 8-hour cortisol level of less than 50% of baseline but 1.4 µg/dL or greater (25% of dogs).

Dexamethasone resistance, in which none of the above criteria is met, occurs in 40% of PDH cases.

Functional adrenal tumor (FAT):
Dexamethasone administration has no effect on cortisol levels.

HIGH-DOSE DEXAMETHASONE SUPPRESSION TEST
Differentiates PDH from FAT in cases where none of the criteria for PDH is met with the LDDST.

FAT:
8-hour cortisol level—no suppression of cortisol levels with dexamethasone administration.

PDH:
8-hour cortisol level is less than 50% of baseline cortisol or less than 1.4 µg/dL.

Disseminated Intravascular Coagulation (DIC), Diagnostic Tests

Fibrinogen: increased

Activated partial thromboplastin time (APTT): prolonged

Prothrombin time (PT): prolonged

Platelet count: decreased

Fibrin degradation products (assays for breakdown of fibrin clots): increased

D-Dimer (assays for proteolytic fragment of fibrinogen degradation): increased

Note: D-Dimer has a high negative predictive value. A negative test reliably rules out DIC.

Eosinophil Count

Normal range:
Feline: 0-1000 cells/μL
Canine: 0-1200 cells/μL

Eosinophils:
Elevated (eosinophilia) in: parasitic disorders (hookworm, dirofilariasis, dipetalonemiasis, fleas, filaroides, aelurostrongylosis, roundworms, paragonimiasis), hypersensitivity (flea allergy dermatitis, atopy, food allergy), eosinophilic infiltrative disease (eosinophilic granuloma complex, feline bronchial asthma, eosinophilic gastroenteritis/colitis, pulmonary infiltrates with eosinophils [dogs], hypereosinophilic syndrome), infectious diseases (toxoplasmosis, suppurative processes), neoplasia (eosinophilic leukemia, mast cell neoplasia, lymphoma, myeloproliferative disorders, solid tumors), hypoadrenocorticism, pregnancy

Decreased (eosinopenia) in: stress, hyperadrenocorticism, glucocorticoid therapy

Erythrocyte Count (Red Blood Cell [RBC] Count)

Normal range:
Feline: 5.92-9.93 10^6/μL
Canine: 4.8-9.3 10^6/μL

Elevated in: dehydration, splenic contraction, polycythemia

Decreased in:
Regenerative anemias
    Acute and chronic hemorrhage
        Gastrointestinal hemorrhage
            Ulcer disease
            Neoplasia

Trauma
Coagulopathies
Ectoparasites (fleas, ticks)
Endoparasites (hookworms, coccidia)
Hematuria
Hemolytic anemia
Immune mediated
Oxidant injury (onion, kale, phenothiazines, methylene blue)
Parasitic
Babesiosis
Mycoplasma haemofelis
Infectious
Leptospirosis
Escherichia coli
Microangiopathic
Dirofilariasis
Vascular neoplasia
Vasculitis
Disseminated intravascular coagulation (DIC)
Nonregenerative anemias
Renal failure
Anemia of chronic disease
Inflammatory disease
Infectious disease
Neoplasia
Drugs
Chemotherapeutics
Chloramphenicol
Iron deficiency
Chronic blood loss
Nutritional
Endocrine disease
Hypothyroidism
Hypoadrenocorticism
Hyperestrogenism
Diethylstilbestrol
Estradiol
Sertoli cell tumor
Infectious
Feline leukemia virus (FeLV)
Feline immunodeficiency virus (FIV)
Ehrlichiosis
Idiopathic aplastic anemia
Red cell aplasia

Myeloproliferative disease
Myelophthisis
Hypersplenism
Lead poisoning

Folate

Normal range:
Feline: 13.4-38.0 ng/mL
Canine: 4.0-13 ng/mL
   Usually performed in conjunction with serum cobalamin and trypsin-like immunoreactivity

Elevated in: exocrine pancreatic insufficiency, small intestinal bacterial overgrowth

Decreased in: small intestinal mucosal disease

Fructosamine

Normal range:
Feline and canine: 175-400 μmol/L
   Single sample test that assays mean blood glucose over the previous 1-3 weeks

Elevated: indicates poor glycemic control (hyperglycemia).

Declining or within normal range: indicates improving or adequate glycemic control.

Decreased to below lower end of reference range: suggests that patient has experienced significant periods of hypoglycemia over past 1-3 weeks.

Values within normal range with PU/PD and polyphagia: suggestive of Somogyi phenomenon.

Note: Fructosamine values should not be used to make specific adjustments in insulin dosage.

Gamma Glutamyltransferase (GGT)

Normal range:
Feline: 1-10 U/L
Canine: 1-12 U/L

Elevated: cholestasis—GGT mirrors alkaline phosphatase (intra-hepatic, extrahepatic), drugs (dogs [glucocorticoids]), anticonvulsants (phenobarbital, primidone), hepatocellular disease (generally slight increase)

Note: Cats with hepatic lipidosis tend to have normal to mildly elevated GGT, but greatly elevated alkaline phosphatase levels.

Decreased: spurious (e.g., laboratory error, lipemic sample), hemolysis

Globulin

Normal range:
Feline: 2.3-5.3 g/dL
Canine: 1.6-3.6 g/dL

Elevated in: dehydration (albumin and total protein also elevated), infection (polyclonal gammopathy; chronic pyoderma, pyometra, chronic periodontitis, feline infectious peritonitis [FIP], ehrlichiosis [may cause polyclonal or monoclonal gammopathy], leishmaniasis [may cause polyclonal or monoclonal gammopathy], systemic mycoses, chronic pneumonia, bartonellosis, *Mycoplasma haemofelis* infection, Chagas' disease, babesiosis), immune-mediated disease (polyclonal gammopathy), neoplasia (polyclonal gammopathy [necrotic or draining tumors, lymphomas, mast cell tumors]), neoplasia (monoclonal gammopathy [multiple myeloma, chronic lymphocytic leukemia, lymphoma]), "idiopathic" monoclonal gammopathy

Glucose

Normal range:
Feline: 64-170 mg/dL
Canine: 70-138 mg/dL

Elevated (hyperglycemia) in: diabetes mellitus, stress (cats), hyperadrenocorticism, drugs (glucocorticoids, progestagens, megesterol acetate, thiazide diuretics), parenteral nutrition, dextrose-containing fluids, postprandial, acromegaly (cats), diestrus (bitch), pheochromocytoma (dogs), exocrine pancreatic neoplasia, renal insufficiency, head trauma

Decreased (hypoglycemia) in: hepatic insufficiency (portal caval shunts, chronic fibrosis, cirrhosis), sepsis, prolonged sample storage, iatrogenic (insulin therapy, sulfonylurea therapy), toxicity (ethanol ingestion, ethylene glycol), β-cell tumor (insulinoma), extrapancreatic neoplasia (hepatocellular carcinoma or hepatoma, leiomyosarcoma or leiomyoma, hemangiosarcoma, carcinoma [mammary, salivary, pulmonary], leukemia, plasmacytoma, melanoma), hypoadrenocorticism, hypopituitarism, idiopathic hypoglycemia (neonatal hypoglycemia, juvenile hypoglycemia [toy breeds], hunting dog hypoglycemia), renal failure, exocrine pancreatic neoplasia, glycogen storage diseases, severe polycythemia, prolonged starvation, laboratory error

Glucose Tolerance Test

May be used to differentiate type 1 (insulin-dependent) from type 2 (non–insulin-dependent) diabetes mellitus in cats (all dogs are considered to have type 1); results inconsistent; not usually done.

Glycosylated Hemoglobin

Assays measure mean blood glucose over the life span of erythrocytes (3-4 months); in dogs, values between 4% and 6% are associated with adequate glycemic control; used less often than fructosamine.

Heartworm Antibody, Feline

Should be interpreted in conjunction with a feline heartworm antigen test.

Should be interpreted in light of clinical, clinicopathologic, and radiographic signs.

Negative test suggests no exposure to *Dirofilaria immitis* and helps to rule out.

Positive supports prior exposure, but does not confirm active infection.

Heartworm Antigen, Canine

Negative test implies no infection.

Positive test supports active infection.

Sample hemolysis may cause false-positive result.

Low worm burden may cause false-negative result.

May remain positive for up to 16 weeks after successful adulticide therapy.

Heartworm Antigen, Feline

Should be interpreted in conjunction with a feline heartworm antibody test.

Negative test is not useful; may still be positive.

Positive test is highly specific; infection is likely.

Should be interpreted in light of clinical, clinicopathologic, and radiographic signs.

Sample hemolysis may cause false-positive result.

Low worm burden or male unisex infection will cause false-negative result.

Hematocrit (Packed Cell Volume, PCV)

Normal range:
Feline: 29%-48%
Canine: 36%-60%

Increased in: dehydration (total protein also increased), polycythemia, splenic contracture

Decreased in: anemia (for more detailed list, see Erythrocyte Count); color of plasma in spun-down hematocrit tube can help determine if icterus (yellow) or intravascular hemolysis (red) is present; buffy coat: may see microfilaria if patient has heartworm disease; mast cells in systemic mastocytosis

Hemoglobin

Hemoglobin concentrations are usually proportional to hematocrit except in rare cases where hemoglobin synthesis defects stimulate polycythemia.

Hemolysis, Prevention in Laboratory Samples

STEPS TO PREVENT HEMOLYSIS:
   Fasted patient: lipemia increases red cell fragility.
   Minimize negative pressure (may cause vein to flutter
      against needle, crushing red cells).
      Reposition needle deeper, or slightly rotate to move
         bevel of needle away from vessel wall.
      Resist tendency to increase vacuum by using more
         negative force; "milk" the vein.
      Use vacuum tubes and needles instead of syringes.
      Remove needle and specimen tube stopper, and transfer
         sample directly into open tube.
      Aspirate small amount of air from tube to reestablish
         negative pressure to prevent tops from coming off in
         transit.

Immunoassays

   **Assays that detect all immunoglobulins to a specific
   antigen in a serum sample:**
      Complement fixation
      Hemagglutination inhibition
      Serum neutralization
      Agglutination assay
   **Assays that may be used to detect specific
   immunoglobulins (IgG, IgM, IgA) to antigens in
   a serum sample:**
      Enzyme-linked immunosorbent assay (ELISA)
      Western blot immunoassay
IgM usually first immunoglobulin produced; may indicate recent infection and more likely to be active infection rather than just previous exposure.

Production of immunoglobulin shifts to IgG and/or IgA in days to weeks; indicates more chronic infection and possibly exposure without active disease.

Demonstrating a rising titer with paired samples may be needed to document active infection.

Insulin

Normal range:
Feline and canine: 15-35 µIU/mL

Elevated: normal or elevated insulin concentration in the presence of hypoglycemia is supportive of insulinoma.

Decreased: decreased insulin levels are not a reliable indicator of diabetes mellitus. Patients with insulin-dependent diabetes mellitus (IDDM) should have low insulin and high glucose levels. Insulin levels in non–insulin-dependent diabetes mellitus (NIDDM) are variable.

Iron-Binding Capacity (Total, TIBC)/Ferritin

Decreased TIBC and decreased ferritin: chronic (not acute) blood loss (intestinal ulceration, hookworm anemia, bleeding from neoplasia, etc.)

TIBC normal to increased, ferritin decreased: iron deficiency

TIBC normal to low, ferritin normal to high: anemia of chronic inflammatory disease

Joint Fluid (Arthrocentesis)

Gross appearance: Evaluate for turbidity (cloudiness), viscosity (does it form a long string when allowed to drip from a needle), and color (clear, red or hemorrhagic, yellow); yellow color (xanthochromia) may indicate previous hemorrhage, degenerative, traumatic, or inflammatory disease.

Microscopic examination/cytologic evaluation:
Normal
1-3 mononuclear cells per high-power field (hpf)
Large and small mononuclear cells with numerous vacuoles
    and granules; less than 10% are neutrophils
    (< 1 neutrophil/500 erythrocytes if blood contamination
    has occurred).

Previous hemorrhage
Hemosiderin-laden macrophage, erythrophagia

Chronic degenerative joint disease
0-12% neutrophils

Immune-mediated joint disease (nonerosive)
15%-95% neutrophils

Traumatic
Variable neutrophils
May see hemorrhage

Septic
90%-99% neutrophils
May see microorganisms within cells
Toxic changes in neutrophils

Rheumatoid arthritis (erosive)
20%-80% neutrophils
    Systemic lupus erythematosus (SLE)–induced polyarthritis:
may see LE cells

Lipase

Normal range:
Feline: 10-450 U/L
Canine: 77-695 U/L

Elevated in: most often seen with acute pancreatitis, pancreatic
necrosis, pancreatic neoplasia, enteritis, renal disease, glucocorticoids; rarely elevated with certain neoplasms in the absence of
pancreatitis.

Note: Not very sensitive or specific for pancreatic disease.

Lymphocyte Count

Normal range:
Feline: 1200-8000 cells/μL
Canine: 690-4500 cells/μL

Elevated (lymphocytosis): physiologic or epinephrine induced, postvaccination, leukemia (lymphocytic, lymphoblastic), chronic antigenic stimulation (inflammatory bowel disease, cholangio-hepatitis, ehrlichiosis, Chagas' disease, babesiosis, leishmaniasis, hypoadrenocorticism)

Decreased (lymphopenia): corticosteroid or stress induced, chemotherapy, immunodeficiency (feline leukemia virus [FeLV], feline immunodeficiency virus [FIV]), loss of lymph (chylotho-rax, lymphangiectasia), viral disease (FeLV/FIV, feline infectious peritonitis [FIP], parvovirus, canine distemper, canine infectious hepatitis)

Magnesium (Mg)

Normal range:
Feline: 1.1-2.3 mEq/L
Canine: 1.2-1.9 mEq/L

Increased in: renal failure or insufficiency

Decreased: dietary, gastrointestinal (malabsorption, chronic diarrhea, pancreatitis), renal (glomerular disease, tubular disease), multiple endocrine disorders, sepsis, blood transfusion, parenteral nutrition, drugs (diuretics, amphotericin B)

Mean Corpuscular Volume (MCV)

Normal range:
Feline: 37-61 fL
Canine: 58-79 fL

Elevated (macrocytosis) in: regeneration, feline leukemia, feline immunodeficiency virus (FIV), breed-related characteristics (poodles), dyserythropoiesis (bone marrow disease)

Decreased (microcytosis) in: iron deficiency, portosystemic shunt, polycythemia, breed-related characteristics (Akita, Shar-Pei, Shiba Inu)

Methemoglobinemia

Methemoglobin is the form of hemoglobin in which the heme iron has been oxidized from ferrous (Fe^{2+}) to ferric (Fe^{3+}) and is rendered unable to bind and transport oxygen.

Methemoglobinemia is seen in oxidative damage-induced hemolytic anemias and with rare inherited erythrocyte disorders.

Monocyte Count

Normal range:
Feline: 0-600 cells/µL
Canine: 0-840 cells/µL

Elevated (monocytosis) in: infection (pyometra, abscess, peritonitis, pyothorax, osteomyelitis, prostatitis, *Mycoplasma haemofelis*, blastomycosis, histoplasmosis, *Cryptococcus, Coccidioides,* heartworm disease, other bacteria [e.g., nocardiosis, actinomycosis, mycobacteriosis]), stress or corticosteroid induced, immune-mediated disease (hemolytic anemia, dermatitis, polyarthritis), trauma with severe crushing injury, hemorrhage into tissues or body cavities, neoplasia (tumor necrosis, lymphoma, myelodysplastic disorders, leukemias, myelomonocytic leukemia, monocytic leukemia, myelogenous leukemia)

Myoglobinuria

Brown to dark-red urine with an absence of red blood cells (RBCs) in urine sediment and a positive test for occult blood; seen with generalized muscle disease.

Neutrophil Count

Normal range:
Feline: 2500-8500 cells/μL
Canine: 2060-10600 cells/μL

Elevated (neutrophilia): increased production (infection [bacterial, systemic mycoses, protozoal], inflammation [immune-mediated disease, neoplasia, tissue trauma, tissue necrosis]), demargination (stress, hyperadrenocorticism, glucocorticoids), metabolic (uremia, diabetic ketoacidosis), associated with regenerative anemia (hemolytic anemia, hemorrhagic anemia), chronic granulocytic leukemia

Decreased (neutropenia): decreased production (myelophthisis [myeloproliferative disease, lymphoproliferative disease, metastatic neoplasia], myelofibrosis, drug induced [chemotherapeutics, griseofulvin, chloramphenicol, trimethoprim-sulfa, azathioprine, estrogen, phenylbutazone, phenobarbital], infectious, parvovirus, ehrlichiosis, FIV, FeLV [aplastic anemia, myelodysplasia, panleukopenia-like syndrome], hypersplenism, idiopathic hypoplasia/aplasia [cyclic neutropenia, immune mediated]), increased consumption (bacteremia/septicemia, severe systemic infection, endotoxemia), hypoadrenocorticism, margination

Osmolality

Plasma osmolality is expected to be decreased in primary polydipsia (psychogenic polydipsia).
Plasma osmolality is expected to be increased in primary polyuria (diabetes insipidus, DI).
There may be considerable overlap in values of primary polyuria and polydipsia. However, osmolality of less than 280 mOsm/kg suggests psychogenic polydipsia, whereas osmolality of greater than 280 mOsm/kg suggests central DI, nephrogenic DI, or psychogenic polydipsia.

Packed Cell Volume

See **Hematocrit.**

Parathyroid Hormone (PTH)/Ionized Calcium

Normal range:
PTH:
Feline: 0.0-40.0 pg/mL
Canine: 20.0-130.0 pg/mL

Ionized calcium:
Feline: 1.16-1.34 mmol/L
Canine: 1.24-1.43 mmol/L

Elevated in: primary hyperparathyroidism (elevated ionized calcium and mid- to high elevated PTH), renal or nutritional secondary hyperparathyroidism (normal or decreased ionized calcium and elevated PTH), hypercalcemia of malignancy, vitamin D toxicity, granulomatous inflammatory disease

Decreased in: primary hypoparathyroidism (decreased ionized calcium and low or low-normal PTH)

Phosphorus (P)

Normal range:
Feline: 2.4-8.2 mg/dL
Canine: 2.5-6.0 mg/dL

Elevated in: young, growing animal (also see elevated alkaline phosphatase), reduced glomerular filtration rate (GFR, acute renal failure, chronic renal failure), postrenal obstruction, hyperparathyroidism, hemolysis, intoxication (hypervitaminosis D, jasmine ingestion), hypoparathyroidism, dietary excess, iatrogenic (phosphate enemas, parenteral administration), osteolysis, sample hemolysis/delayed serum separation

Decreased in: primary hyperparathyroidism (also see increased calcium), nutritional secondary hyperparathyroidism, renal tubular acidosis, neoplasia (PTH-like hormone, C-cell thyroid tumors), insulin therapy, diabetic ketoacidosis, Fanconi's syndrome, dietary deficiency, eclampsia, hyperadrenocorticism

Platelet Count

Normal range:
Feline: 200-500 $10^3/\mu$L
Canine: 170-400 $10^3/\mu$L

Elevated in: essential thrombocytosis, rebound thrombocytosis, polycythemia vera

Decreased (see p. 142): decreased production (infectious [retroviruses: feline immunodeficiency virus, feline leukemia virus; *Ehrlichia*]), increased destruction (immune-mediated thrombocytopenia), sequestration (hypersplenism), increased consumption (hemorrhage, disseminated intravascular coagulation), breed idiosyncrasy (King Charles Spaniels [macrothrombocytes], Greyhounds)

Potassium (K)

Normal range:
Feline: 3.4-5.6 g/dL
Canine: 3.6-5.5 g/dL

Elevated in: renal failure (distal renal tubular acidosis, oliguric/anuric), postrenal (obstruction, ruptured bladder), hypoadrenocorticism, acidosis (diabetic ketoacidosis), massive muscle trauma, postischemic reperfusion, dehydration, hypoaldosteronism, drugs (potassium-sparing diuretics, ACE inhibitors, propranolol)

Decreased in: alkalosis, dietary deficiency (feline), potassium-free fluids, bicarbonate administration, drugs (penicillins, amphotericin B, loop diuretics), gastrointestinal fluid loss (potassium rich), hyperadrenocorticism, hyperaldosteronism, insulin therapy, renal (postobstructive diuresis, renal tubular acidosis, dialysis), hypokalemic periodic paralysis (Burmese cat, Pit Bull Terrier), renal failure (chronic polyuria)

Protein, Total (TP)

Normal range:
Feline: 5.2-8.8 g/dL
Canine: 5.0-7.4 g/dL

Elevated in: dehydration (albumin and globulin increased), hyperglobulinemia (chronic inflammation, infection, neoplasia [e.g., multiple myeloma]), spurious (hemolysis, lipemia)

Decreased in: hemorrhage, hypoalbuminemia, liver failure, external plasma loss, gastrointestinal fluid loss, malassimilation, starvation, overhydration, glomerular loss, tumor cachexia

Prothrombin Time (PT)

Normal range:
Feline: 6-11 seconds
Canine: 6-12 seconds

Determines abnormalities in the extrinsic coagulation pathway
Prolonged with deficiencies of factors II, VII, and X
Becomes prolonged before any changes seen in activated coagulation time (ACT) or activated partial thromboplastin time (APTT)

Red Blood Cell (RBC) Count

See **Erythrocyte Count.**

Reticulocyte Count

Elevated reticulocyte count is the best indicator of effective erythropoiesis.
Step 1: Multiply percent reticulocytes by red cell count to determine absolute quantity.
Step 2: Correct for reduced red cell mass; multiply absolute reticulocytes by patient's hematocrit divided by mean species hematocrit to obtain the number of reticulocytes per milliliter.
Step 3: Correct for the effect of erythropoietin on the bone marrow reticulocyte release; divide the number of reticulocytes per milliliter by average number of days that a reticulocyte circulates in peripheral blood at that patient's hematocrit to obtain a corrected absolute reticulocyte count. A corrected absolute reticulocyte count of less than

105,000/mL is indicative of a nonregenerative anemia, whereas strongly regenerative anemias will have a reticulocyte count of greater than 150,000/mL.

Sodium (Na)

Normal range:
Feline: 145-158 mEq/L
Canine: 139-154 mEq/L

Elevated in: dehydration, renal failure, gastrointestinal (GI) fluid loss (Na^+ poor) (vomiting, diarrhea), insensible fluid loss (panting, high ambient temperature, fever), decreased water intake (limited access to water, primary adipsia), hyperaldosteronemia, increased salt intake (oral, intravenous), spurious (evaporation of serum sample)

Decreased in: hypoadrenocorticism, GI fluid loss (Na+ rich) (vomiting, diarrhea), hookworms, renal failure (polyuric), chronic effusions, diuretics, hypotonic fluids, diabetes mellitus, burns, excess antidiuretic hormone (ADH), diet (severe sodium restriction), psychogenic polydipsia, spurious (hyperlipidemia)

Thoracocentesis Fluid

Pyothorax (septic)
Extremely high nucleated cell counts (> 50,000/µL)
Primarily degenerate neutrophils and macrophages
Bacteria seen in white blood cells (WBCs)
Penetrating wounds, foreign body (grass awns), extension of
    bacterial pneumonia

Nonseptic
Moderate nucleated cell counts (> 5000/µL)
Neutrophils, macrophages, eosinophils, lymphocytes
Feline infectious peritonitis (FIP), neoplasia, diaphragmatic
    hernia, lung lobe torsion

Chylous effusion
Low to moderate nucleated cell counts (400-10,000/µL)
Predominant cell type is small lymphocyte; also neutrophils
    and macrophages.

Triglyceride concentration of pleural fluid is greater than that of serum.
Idiopathic
Congenital
Secondary to neoplasia, trauma, cardiac disease, pericardial disease, dirofilariasis, lung lobe torsion, and diaphragmatic hernia

Hemorrhagic effusion
Trauma
Coagulopathy
Neoplasia
Lung lobe torsion

Transudates and modified transudates
Protein concentrations less than 2.5-3.0 g/dL
Low nucleated cell count (< 500-1000/μL)
Macrophages, lymphocytes, mesothelial cells
Right-sided heart failure, pericardial disease, hypoalbuminemia, neoplasia, diaphragmatic hernia

Note:
   Neoplastic cells may or may not be present in effusions caused by neoplastic processes.

Thrombocyte Count

See **Platelet Count.**

Thyroid Function Tests

Total T_4 (Thyroxine, Tetraiodothyronine):
Measures free T_4 and protein-bound T_4.
Below-normal values suggest hypothyroidism (dogs).
Above-normal values in cats are likely caused by hyperthyroidism.
Below-normal values are also seen with underlying illness (sick, euthyroid).

Free T_4 (FT_4):
Below-normal values suggest hypothyroidism (dogs).
Above-normal values in cats are likely caused by hyperthyroidism.

Not as affected by the suppressive effects of concurrent illness
as total T_4.
Modified equilibrium dialysis assay is not affected by
circulating antithyroid hormone antibodies and therefore is
the preferred assay for fT_4.

Thyroid-stimulating hormone (TSH) concentration:
Must be interpreted in conjunction with serum T_4 and fT_4.
Low value for serum T_4 and fT_4 with a high TSH supports
diagnosis of hypothyroidism.
Normal T_4 and fT_4 and normal TSH rule out hypothyroidism.

TSH and thyroid-releasing hormone (TRH) stimulation tests:
Used to differentiate hypothyroidism from euthyroid sick
syndrome.
These tests are not typically done because of availability and
expense of reagents.

T_3 (3,5,3'-triiodothyronine) concentration:
Poor indicator of thyroid function in dogs and cats; not
recommended.

Tests for lymphocytic thyroiditis:
Autoantibodies to circulating thyroid hormone (T_4 and T_3) and
thyroglobulin (Tg) correlate with lymphocytic thyroiditis.
Tg autoantibodies may be present when T_4 and T_3 are not;
therefore, test for Tg autoantibodies is considered the better
screening test.
Provides no information about the severity of disease or the
extent of thyroid gland involvement.
Hypothyroid dogs may be negative, and euthyroid dogs may
have Tg autoantibodies.
May be used as a prebreeding screening test in breeding dogs.

Toxoplasmosis Antibody Titer

Positive titer indicates exposure, but not necessarily active
infection.
Positive IgM titer greater than 1:256 is consistent with
active infection, especially with typical clinical signs.
Fourfold rise in IgG titer of paired samples 2 to 3 weeks
apart also supports active infection.

Triglycerides

Normal range:
Feline: 25-160 mg/dL
Canine: 29-291 mg/dL

Elevated in: postprandial, familial triglyceridemia (Miniature Schnauzer, other breeds), hyperchylomicronemia of cats (also observed in dogs), lipoprotein lipase deficiency (cat), endocrine disorders (hypothyroidism, hyperadrenocorticism, diabetes mellitus), nephrotic syndrome, pancreatitis, cholestasis, drugs (glucocorticoids, megestrol acetate)

Decreased in: not clearly associated with any disease; severe malabsorptive protein-losing enteropathy, hyperthyroidism

Trypsinogen-Like Immunoreactivity (TLI)
Pancreatic Lipase Immunoreactivity (PLI)

Normal range:
TLI:
Feline: 12.0-82.0 µg/L
Canine: 5.0-35.0 µg/L

PLI:
Feline: 2.0-6.8 µg/L
Canine: 0-200 µg/L
     Low TLI values (< 2.5 µg/L for dogs and < 8.0 µg/L for cats) are diagnostic for exocrine pancreatic insufficiency; values between 2.5 and 5.0 µg/L for dogs and 8.0 and 12.0 µg/L for cats are considered equivocal, and the assay should be repeated in 1 month.
     High values for TLI are supportive of a diagnosis of acute or chronic pancreatitis.
     Elevated values for PLI (> 12 µg/L for cats and > 400 µg/L for dogs) are consistent with a diagnosis of pancreatitis.
     Patients must be fasted at least 12 hours.

Note: These tests are species specific, and samples must be labeled "dog" or "cat" so that the test can be performed correctly.

Urinalysis

APPEARANCE

Color

Yellow (normal): may be dark amber when concentrated and pale to colorless when dilute. However, color does not always correlate with concentration.

Red or reddish-brown: hematuria, hemoglobinuria, myoglobinuria

Dark brown or black: methemoglobinuria

Yellow-brown to yellow-green: concentrated sample, bilirubinuria, *Pseudomonas* infection

Orange: bilirubinuria

Turbidity

Normally clear; cloudy urine may contain cellular material, crystals, and mucus.

Odor

Excess ammonia odor may be detectable in urine infected with urease-producing bacteria.

SPECIFIC GRAVITY

Normal
Feline: 1.025-1.060
Canine: 1.020-1.050

Isosthenuria (1.008-1.012)
Renal failure
Rare cases of polydipsia

Hyposthenuria (< 1.008)
Polydipsia/polyuria
Diabetes insipidus

CHEMICAL PROPERTIES

pH

Normal: 5.5-7.5 (feline and canine)

Causes of acidic urine: meat-based diet, administration of acidifying agents (e.g., D,L-methionine, NH_4Cl), metabolic acidosis, respiratory acidosis, protein catabolic states, chloride depletion

Causes of alkaline urine: vegetable-based diet, administration of alkalinizing agents (e.g., $NaHCO_3$, citrate), urinary tract infection by urease-producing bacteria, postprandial alkaline tide, metabolic alkalosis, respiratory alkalosis, renal tubular acidosis (distal tubule)

Protein

Normal: 0-30 mg/dL
Commonly used dipsticks are more sensitive to albumin than globulin.
Increased with glomerular or inflammatory disease

Glucose
Appears in urine if the renal threshold is exceeded
Diabetes mellitus, proximal renal tubular diseases

Ketones
Beta-hydroxybutyrate, acetoacetate, acetone
Elevated in diabetes ketoacidosis, starvation, prolonged fasting, glycogen storage disease, low-carbohydrate diet, persistent fever, persistent hypoglycemia

Occult Blood
Does not differentiate among erythrocytes (RBCs), hemoglobin, and myoglobin
Always interpreted in light of urine sediment (evaluation for RBCs)
    Erythrocytes—hematuria
    Hemoglobin—hemolysis
    Myoglobin—rhabdomyolysis

Bilirubin
Detectable in urine before it is elevated in serum
May be found in trace amounts in concentrated samples, especially in intact males
Bilirubinuria seen in hemolysis, liver disease, extrahepatic obstruction, fever, starvation

Urobilinogen
Presence indicates normal enterohepatic bilirubin circulation.

URINARY SEDIMENT EXAMINATION

Red Blood Cells (RBCs)
Normally, zero to occasional RBCs; excessive RBCs termed *hematuria* (see p. 34)

White Blood Cells (WBCs)
Normally, zero to occasional WBCs
Excessive WBCs termed *pyuria;* indicates urinary tract infection but does not localize the site of infection

Epithelial Cells

Squamous and transitional cells, little diagnostic significance

Increased transitional cells may be seen with infection, neoplasia, and irritation of the urinary tract.

Casts

Cylindrical molds of renal tubules composed of aggregated proteins or cells that localize disease to the kidney.

Occasional hyaline or granular cast may be normal; cellular casts are always abnormal.

> *Hyaline casts:* protein precipitates (Tamm-Horsfall mucoprotein and albumin); seen with proteinuric renal disease (glomerulonephritis, amyloidosis), small numbers with fever and exercise
>
> *Granular casts:* degeneration of cells in casts or precipitation of filtered plasma proteins; suggest ischemic or nephrotoxic renal tubular injury
>
> *Cellular casts:* WBC casts (pyelonephritis), RBC casts (fragile, rare in dogs and cats), renal epithelial cell casts (acute tubular necrosis or pyelonephritis)
>
> *Fatty casts:* lipid granules (nephrotic syndrome or diabetes mellitus)
>
> *Waxy casts:* final stage of degeneration of granular casts (suggest intrarenal stasis)
>
> *Organisms:* small numbers of bacteria may contaminate voided or catheterized samples, but usually not enough to be seen in urine sediment unless sample is allowed to incubate. Presence of large numbers of bacteria in sediment suggests urinary tract infection. Yeast and fungal hyphae usually are contaminants.

Crystals

Usually of little diagnostic value; typically found in normal urine.

> Acidic urine may contain urate, calcium oxalate, and cystine crystals.
>
> Alkaline urine may contain struvite, calcium phosphate, calcium carbonate, amorphous phosphate, and ammonium biurate crystals.
>
> Bilirubin crystals may be seen with concentrated samples or with bilirubinuria.
>
> Urate crystals may be seen in Dalmatians and with liver disease or portosystemic shunts.
>
> Struvite crystals are seen in cats with idiopathic lower urinary tract disease, dogs, and cats with struvite urolithiasis.

Calcium oxalate in oliguric acute renal failure (ARF) suggests ethylene glycol intoxication.

Cystine crystals, when abnormal, suggest cystinuria.

Other Findings in Sediment
Sperm in intact male dogs
Parasite ova; *Dioctophyma renale, Capillaria plica*
Microfilariae
Lipid droplets (diabetes mellitus, nephrotic syndrome, in cats with degeneration of lipid-laden tubular cells)

Common Bacteria Seen in Urinary Tract Infections
Escherichia coli
Proteus spp.
Staphylococcus spp.
Pasteurella multocida
Enterobacter spp.
Klebsiella spp.
Pseudomonas aeruginosa

Urine Cortisol/Creatinine Ratio

Very sensitive, but not very specific test for hyperadrenocorticism.

Good test to rule out hyperadrenocorticism, but not to diagnose.

von Willebrand's Factor

Variable degrees of expression of factor for von Willebrand's disease (vWD), a common, inherited hemostatic disorder (rare in cats).

Dogs with levels less than 30% are prone to spontaneous bleeding (e.g., epistaxis).

Classification of vWD in dogs:

Type I: low concentration of normal von Willebrand's factor

Type II: low-normal concentration of abnormal von Willebrand's factor

Type III: absence of von Willebrand's factor

Hemostatic screening tests usually are normal in dogs with vWD.

Buccal mucosal bleeding time is the exception—best screening test.

White Blood Cell (WBC) Count

Normal range:
Feline: 3.5-16.0 $10^3/\mu L$
Canine: 4.0-15.5 $10^3/\mu L$

Elevated in: infection (bacterial, systemic mycoses), physiologic leukocytosis, metabolic (stress, glucocorticoids), inflammation (immune-mediated disease, neoplasia, tissue trauma, tissue necrosis), leukemia, associated with responsive anemia (hemorrhagic anemia, hemolytic anemia)

Decreased in: decreased production, increased consumption, neutropenia secondary to phenobarbital administration

Index

A

Abdomen
    disorders, causes. *See* Acute abdomen disorders
    free fluid, 2
    free gas, 2
Abdominal distension, 2-3
    fat, impact, 3
    feces, impact, 3
    fluid, impact, 2
    gas, impact, 2
Abdominal effusions/ascites, 3-4
    blood, impact, 4
Abdominal musculature. *See* Weakened abdominal musculature
Abdominal pain. *See* Acute abdominal pain
Acetylcholine receptor antibody, 238
Acquired coagulopathy, 137
    differential diagnosis, 137
Acquired late-onset conductive deafness, 20
Acquired late-onset sensorineural deafness, 20
Acromegaly, 100-101
    clinical findings. *See* Cats; Dogs
ACTH. See Adrenocorticotropic hormone
Activated coagulation time (ACT), 238
Activated partial thromboplastin time (APTT), 238
Acute abdomen disorders, causes, 123-124
Acute abdominal pain, 4-5
Acute blindness, 209-210
    differential diagnosis. *See* Cats; Dogs
Acute diarrhea, 21
    diet, impact, 21
    infectious impact, 21
    parasites, impact, 21
Acute pancreatitis, clinical findings, 178-179
Acute renal failure, 9
    causes. *See* Cats; Dogs
Adrenal tumors, 101-102
    differential diagnosis, 101-102
    functional adrenomedullary tumor, 102
Adrenocorticotropic hormone (ACTH). *See* Endogenous ACTH
    stimulation tests, 239
Aggressive behavior, 5-6
Alanine aminotransferase (ALT // SGPT), 240
Albumin, 240
Alimentary disorders, impact. *See* Regurgitation
Alimentary tract lesion, 32-33. *See also* Extraalimentary tract lesion
Alkaline phosphatase. *See* Serum alkaline phosphatase